The Adjustment Myth

How Chiropractic Falls
Short of Its Promises

The HealthSpan Institute

The Adjustment Myth:
How Chiropractic Falls Short of Its Promises

ISBN: 9798327810693

Printed in the United States of America

Contents

Chapter 5:
The Efficacy Debate:
Does Chiropractic Really Work?

Chapter 6:
Risks and Concerns in Chiropractic Care

Chapter 7:
The Alternatives:
Evidence-Based Approaches to Musculoskeletal Health

Chapter 8:
Navigating the Chiropractic Landscape

Chapter 9:
Conclusion

Chapter 1: Introduction

A Brief History of Chiropractic and Its Rise in Popularity

The story of chiropractic begins in the late 19th century with Daniel David Palmer, a magnetic healer from Iowa [1]. In 1895, Palmer claimed to have restored the hearing of a janitor named Harvey Lillard by adjusting a misaligned vertebra in his spine [2]. This event marked the birth of chiropractic, a term derived from the Greek words "cheir" (hand) and "praktos" (done), reflecting the manual nature of the therapy [1].

Palmer's theory revolved around the concept of "subluxation," which he described as misalignments of the vertebrae causing nerve interference and leading to various health problems [1]. He believed that correcting these subluxations through spinal adjustments could restore proper nerve function and allow the body to heal itself [2]. In 1897, Palmer founded the Palmer School of Cure, later known as the Palmer School of Chiropractic, in Davenport, Iowa, to teach his methods to others [2].

As chiropractic grew, it faced significant challenges and opposition from the medical establishment [2]. In the early 20th century, chiropractors were often arrested for practicing medicine without a license, as their approach was seen as unscientific and unproven [3]. Despite this, chiropractic continued to gain popularity, particularly during the 1918 influenza pandemic, as many patients turned to alternative therapies in the face of mainstream medicine's limitations [2].

Over time, chiropractic began to establish itself as a distinct profession [2]. In 1963, the National Board of Chiropractic Examiners was formed to standardize education and licensing requirements [2]. By the 1970s, most states had recognized chiropractic as a licensed profession, and insurance companies began to cover chiropractic services [2].

The rise of chiropractic can be attributed to several factors [2]. First, it offered a non-invasive, drug-free approach to health care that appealed to many people who were dissatisfied with conventional medicine [2]. Second, chiropractors often provided personalized, hands-on care that patients found comforting and reassuring [2]. Third, the profession's emphasis on wellness and prevention resonated with a growing interest in holistic health and alternative therapies [2].

However, as chiropractic gained acceptance, it also faced increased scrutiny from the scientific community [4]. Many of its core beliefs, such as the subluxation theory, have been challenged by modern research [4]. Some studies have suggested that while chiropractic may be effective for certain musculoskeletal conditions, such as low back pain, its efficacy for other health issues remains questionable [4].

Despite these challenges, chiropractic has continued to thrive [2]. Today, it is the largest alternative health profession in the United States, with over 70,000 licensed practitioners [2]. Chiropractic services are now covered by most major health insurance plans, and many hospitals and health centers have integrated chiropractors into their multidisciplinary teams [2].

As the profession evolves, it faces ongoing debates about its scope of practice, its integration with mainstream medicine, and the need for more rigorous scientific research to support its claims [3]. Some chiropractors have embraced evidence-based practices and interdisciplinary collaboration, while others continue to adhere to traditional philosophies and techniques [3].

The history of chiropractic is a complex tapestry woven from threads of innovation, controversy, and perseverance [3]. As the profession moves forward, it must grapple with its past while charting a course toward a future grounded in science, ethics, and patient-centered care [3].

References

1. Palmer, D. D. (1910). The Chiropractor's Adjuster: The Science, Art, and Philosophy of Chiropractic. Portland Printing House.
2. Wardwell, W. I. (1992). Chiropractic: History and Evolution of a New Profession. Mosby Year Book.
3. Johnson, C. (2010). Reflecting on 115 years: the chiropractic profession's philosophical path. Journal of Chiropractic Humanities, 17(1), 1-5.
4. Ernst, E. (2008). Chiropractic: a critical evaluation. Journal of Pain and Symptom Management, 35(5), 544-562.

Chiropractic Care: Promises, Scientific Shortcomings, and the Quest for Long-Term Relief

Chiropractic care has long been touted as a natural, non-invasive solution to a wide range of health problems, from chronic back pain to headaches and even asthma [1]. Proponents of chiropractic often claim that by manipulating the spine and correcting misalignments, known as subluxations, they can alleviate pain, improve function, and promote overall well-being [2]. However, despite these promises, the scientific evidence supporting the efficacy of chiropractic care remains limited and controversial [3].

At the heart of the debate surrounding chiropractic lies the concept of subluxation, which has been a central tenet of the profession since its inception [4]. According to traditional chiropractic theory, subluxations interfere with the body's innate intelligence, disrupting the flow of nerve energy and leading to disease [5]. While this idea may have held sway in the early days of chiropractic, modern scientific understanding of the human body has largely discredited the notion of innate intelligence and the significance of subluxations [6].

Numerous studies have sought to evaluate the effectiveness of chiropractic care for various conditions, with mixed results [7]. While some research suggests that chiropractic manipulation may provide short-term relief for certain types of low back pain, neck pain, and headaches, the evidence for its long-term benefits is less convincing [8]. Moreover, the mechanisms by which chiropractic interventions might work remain poorly understood, and the studies that do show positive outcomes often suffer from methodological limitations, such as small sample sizes, lack of control groups, and reliance on subjective measures of pain [9].

One of the key challenges in assessing the efficacy of chiropractic care is the lack of standardization within the profession [10]. Chiropractic techniques and philosophies vary widely among practitioners, ranging from those who adhere strictly to traditional subluxation-based models to those who incorporate elements of physical therapy, rehabilitation, and evidence-based practice [11]. This diversity makes it difficult to draw broad conclusions about the effectiveness of chiropractic as a whole, as the quality and approach of individual practitioners can vary significantly [12].

Another concern surrounding chiropractic care is the potential for adverse events, particularly when it comes to cervical spine manipulation [13]. While serious complications are rare, there have been documented cases of stroke, vertebral artery dissection, and other neurological injuries following chiropractic neck adjustments [14]. The risk of these events, although small, underscores the need for chiropractors to thoroughly screen patients, obtain informed consent, and employ techniques that minimize the potential for harm [15].

Perhaps most troubling is the tendency of some chiropractors to make bold claims about their ability to treat conditions that lie outside the musculoskeletal realm, such as asthma, allergies, and even cancer [16]. These claims are often based on anecdotal evidence or outdated theories rather than rigorous scientific research, and they can lead patients to delay or forego necessary medical treatment in favor of chiropractic care [17].

Despite these concerns, chiropractic remains a popular choice for many individuals seeking relief from pain and other symptoms [18]. The appeal of chiropractic may lie in its non-invasive, drug-free approach, as well as the personalized attention and hands-on care that patients often receive from their chiropractors [19]. However, it is essential for patients to approach chiropractic with a critical eye, to ask questions about the evidence behind their practitioner's techniques, and to be wary of promises that seem too good to be true [20].

In conclusion, while chiropractic care may offer temporary relief for some musculoskeletal conditions, its scientific foundations remain shaky, and its long-term benefits are uncertain. As the profession continues to evolve, it will be important for chiropractors to embrace evidence-based practices, to collaborate with other healthcare providers, and to prioritize patient safety and well-being over adherence to outdated dogmas. Only by holding itself to the highest standards of scientific rigor and ethical practice can chiropractic hope to secure a legitimate place in the modern healthcare landscape.

References

1. Ernst, E. (2008). Chiropractic: a critical evaluation. Journal of Pain and Symptom Management, 35(5), 544-562.
2. Keating, J. C., Jr, Charlton, K. H., Grod, J. P., Perle, S. M., Sikorski, D., & Winterstein, J. F. (2005). Subluxation: dogma or science? Chiropractic & Osteopathy, 13, 17.
3. Posadzki, P., & Ernst, E. (2011). Spinal manipulation: an update of a systematic review of systematic reviews. The New Zealand Medical Journal, 124(1340), 55-71.
4. Mirtz, T. A., Morgan, L., Wyatt, L. H., & Greene, L. (2009). An epidemiological examination of the subluxation construct using Hill's criteria of causation. Chiropractic & Osteopathy, 17, 13.
5. Keating, J. C., Jr. (2003). Several pathways in the evolution of chiropractic manipulation. Journal of Manipulative and Physiological Therapeutics, 26(5), 300-321.
6. Homola, S. (2006). Chiropractic: history and overview of theories and methods. Clinical Orthopaedics and Related Research, 444, 236-242.
7. Rubinstein, S. M., van Middelkoop, M., Assendelft, W. J., de Boer, M. R., & van Tulder, M. W. (2011). Spinal manipulative therapy for chronic low-back pain: an update of a Cochrane review. Spine, 36(13), E825-E846.
8. Bronfort, G., Haas, M., Evans, R., Leininger, B., & Triano, J. (2010). Effectiveness of manual therapies: the UK evidence report. Chiropractic & Osteopathy, 18, 3.
9. Ernst, E., & Canter, P. H. (2006). A systematic review of systematic reviews of spinal manipulation. Journal of the Royal Society of Medicine, 99(4), 192-196.
10. Villanueva-Russell, Y. (2011). Caught in the crosshairs: identity and cultural authority within chiropractic. Social Science & Medicine, 72(11), 1826-1837.
11. McGregor, M., Puhl, A. A., Reinhart, C., Injeyan, H. S., & Soave, D. (2014). Differentiating intraprofessional attitudes toward paradigms in health care delivery among chiropractic factions: results from a randomly sampled survey. BMC Complementary and Alternative Medicine, 14, 51.
12. Kaptchuk, T. J., & Eisenberg, D. M. (1998). Chiropractic: origins, controversies, and contributions. Archives of Internal Medicine, 158(20), 2215-2224.
13. Ernst, E. (2007). Adverse effects of spinal manipulation: a systematic review. Journal of the Royal Society of Medicine, 100(7), 330-338.
14. Cassidy, J. D., Boyle, E., Côté, P., He, Y., Hogg-Johnson, S., Silver, F. L., & Bondy, S. J. (2008). Risk of vertebrobasilar stroke and chiropractic care: results of a population-based case-control and case-crossover study. Spine, 33(4 Suppl), S176-S183.
15. Haldeman, S., Kohlbeck, F. J., & McGregor, M. (1999). Risk factors and precipitating neck movements causing vertebrobasilar artery dissection after cervical trauma and spinal manipulation. Spine, 24(8), 785-794.
16. Homola, S. (2010). Real orthopaedic subluxations versus imaginary chiropractic subluxations. Focus on Alternative and Complementary Therapies, 15(4), 284-287.

17. Posadzki, P., & Ernst, E. (2013). Spinal manipulation: a systematic review of sham-controlled, double-blind, randomized clinical trials. Journal of Pain and Symptom Management, 46(4), 605-612.

18. Barnes, P. M., Bloom, B., & Nahin, R. L. (2008). Complementary and alternative medicine use among adults and children: United States, 2007. National Health Statistics Reports, (12), 1-23.

19. Coulter, I. D., & Shekelle, P. G. (2005). Chiropractic in North America: a descriptive analysis. Journal of Manipulative and Physiological Therapeutics, 28(2), 83-89.

20. Haynes, M. J., Vincent, K., Fischhoff, C., Bremner, A. P., Lanlo, O., & Hankey, G. J. (2012). Assessing the risk of stroke from neck manipulation: a systematic review. International Journal of Clinical Practice, 66(10), 940-947.

Chapter 2:
The Origins of Chiropractic

D.D. Palmer: The Enigmatic Founder of Chiropractic

The story of chiropractic begins with a charismatic and controversial figure named Daniel David Palmer. Born in 1845 in Port Perry, Ontario, Canada, Palmer's early life was marked by a series of eclectic pursuits and a fascination with the healing arts [1]. He worked as a beekeeper, school teacher, and grocery store owner before turning his attention to alternative medicine in the late 1800s [2].

Palmer's interest in healing was sparked by his own experiences with chronic health problems, including headaches and deafness [3]. Dissatisfied with the conventional medical treatments of his day, he began to explore various alternative therapies, such as magnetic healing, spiritual healing, and osteopathy [4]. It was against this backdrop of personal experimentation and intellectual curiosity that Palmer would make the discovery that would change the course of his life and give birth to a new profession.

The pivotal moment in chiropractic history occurred on September 18, 1895, when Palmer encountered a janitor named Harvey Lillard in his office building in Davenport, Iowa [5]. Lillard had been deaf for 17 years, and Palmer noticed a prominent lump on his back. According to Palmer's account, he asked Lillard to lie down on a bench and proceeded to manipulate the lump, which he believed to be a misaligned vertebra [6]. Lillard reportedly heard a popping sound and immediately regained his hearing [7].

Convinced that he had discovered a new healing principle, Palmer began to develop his theory of chiropractic. He postulated that misalignments of the spine, which he called "subluxations," could interfere with the body's innate intelligence, leading to a wide range of health problems [8]. By correcting these subluxations through spinal adjustments, Palmer believed that he could restore the flow of nerve energy and allow the body to heal itself [9].

Word of Palmer's newfound healing technique spread quickly, and he soon found himself treating a growing number of patients [10]. In 1897, he established the Palmer School of Cure, later known as the Palmer School of Chiropractic, to teach his methods to others [11]. The school's first graduate was Palmer's own son, Bartlett Joshua Palmer, who would go on to play a significant role in the development and promotion of chiropractic [12].

As chiropractic gained popularity, Palmer faced numerous challenges and controversies. He was repeatedly arrested and jailed for practicing medicine without a license, as the medical establishment viewed his methods with suspicion and hostility [13]. Palmer also engaged in bitter disputes with his son, B.J., over the direction and control of the chiropractic school [14].

Despite these difficulties, Palmer remained a tireless advocate for chiropractic until his death in 1913 [15]. He wrote extensively on his theories and techniques, publishing several books and pamphlets, including "The Chiropractor's Adjuster" and "The Science, Art, and Philosophy of Chiropractic" [16]. Although some of his ideas, such as the concept of innate intelligence, have been largely discredited by modern science, his emphasis on the importance of the nervous system and the spine in overall health continues to influence chiropractic practice today [17].

Palmer's legacy is a complex one, marked by both innovation and controversy. Some view him as a visionary healer who challenged the orthodoxy of his time and pioneered a new approach to healthcare [18]. Others see him as a misguided and unscientific practitioner who promoted a system based on pseudoscience and anecdotal evidence [19]. Regardless of one's perspective, there is no denying the profound impact that D.D. Palmer had on the development of chiropractic and the broader field of alternative medicine.

As the chiropractic profession continues to evolve and grapple with its identity and place in the modern healthcare landscape, it is important to understand and critically examine its origins. By exploring the life and work of D.D. Palmer, we can gain insights into the foundational principles and practices of chiropractic, as well as the challenges and controversies that have shaped its history. Only by confronting this complex legacy can the profession hope to move forward in a way that is grounded in science, evidence, and a commitment to patient well-being.

References

1. Keating, J. C., Jr. (1997). D. D. Palmer: The origins of the chiropractic profession. Journal of Chiropractic Humanities, 7, 3-13.
2. Peterson, D., & Wiese, G. (1995). Chiropractic: An Illustrated History. Mosby-Year Book.
3. Gielow, V. (1981). Old Dad Chiro: A Biography of D. D. Palmer, Founder of Chiropractic. W.B. Conkey Company.
4. Wardwell, W. I. (1992). Chiropractic: History and Evolution of a New Profession. Mosby-Year Book.
5. Palmer, D. D. (1910). The Chiropractor's Adjuster: The Science, Art, and Philosophy of Chiropractic. Portland Printing House.
6. Colquhoun, D., & Novella, S. P. (2013). Acupuncture is theatrical placebo. Anesthesia & Analgesia, 116(6), 1360-1363.
7. Palmer, B. J. (1949). The Bigness of the Fellow Within. Palmer School of Chiropractic.
8. Keating, J. C., Jr. (2003). Several pathways in the evolution of chiropractic manipulation. Journal of Manipulative and Physiological Therapeutics, 26(5), 300-321.
9. Palmer, D. D. (1914). The Chiropractor. Beacon Light Printing Company.
10. Moore, J. S. (1993). Chiropractic in America: The History of a Medical Alternative. Johns Hopkins University Press.
11. Rehm, W. S. (1986). Legally defensible: Chiropractic in the courtroom and after, 1907. Chiropractic History, 6(1), 51-55.
12. Keating, J. C., Jr. (1995). D. D. Palmer's forgotten theories of chiropractic. Association for the History of Chiropractic.
13. Turner, C. (1931). The Rise of Chiropractic. Powell Publishing Company.
14. Gibbons, R. W. (1994). Forgotten parameters of general practice: The chiropractic obstetrician. Chiropractic History, 14(1), 27-33.
15. Keating, J. C., Jr. (1997). Chiropractic: science and antiscience and pseudoscience side by side. Skeptical Inquirer, 21(4), 37-43.
16. Palmer, D. D. (1900). The Chiropractor's Adjuster: Text-Book of the Science, Art and Philosophy of Chiropractic for Students and Practitioners. Self-published.
17. Leach, R. A. (2004). The Chiropractic Theories: A Textbook of Scientific Research. Lippincott Williams & Wilkins.
18. Senzon, S. A. (2010). Chiropractic and Energy Medicine: A Shared History. Journal of Chiropractic Humanities, 17(1), 27-54.
19. Ernst, E. (2008). Chiropractic: a critical evaluation. Journal of Pain and Symptom Management, 35(5), 544-562.

Early Controversies and Conflicts with Mainstream Medicine

As chiropractic began to gain traction in the early 20th century, it quickly found itself at odds with the established medical community. The relationship between chiropractors and medical doctors was fraught with tension, mistrust, and often outright hostility [1]. This conflict was fueled by a combination of philosophical differences, professional rivalries, and legal battles that would shape the course of chiropractic's development for decades to come.

At the heart of the conflict was a fundamental disagreement about the nature of disease and the role of the physician. Chiropractors, led by the charismatic and uncompromising D.D. Palmer, espoused a vitalistic philosophy that emphasized the body's innate ability to heal itself [2]. They believed that misalignments of the spine, known as subluxations, could interfere with the flow of "innate intelligence" and lead to a wide range of health problems [3]. By contrast, the medical establishment, which was undergoing a period of rapid scientific advancement and professionalization, viewed disease as the result of specific, identifiable causes that could be addressed through evidence-based interventions [4].

Medical doctors were deeply skeptical of chiropractic's theoretical foundations and saw the practice as a threat to public health [5]. They accused chiropractors of practicing medicine without proper training or licensure and of misleading the public with unsubstantiated claims [6]. In response, chiropractors argued that their approach was a distinct and complementary form of healthcare that should be regulated separately from medicine [7].

The conflict between chiropractors and medical doctors played out in the legal arena, as well as in the court of public opinion. In the early 1900s, chiropractors faced numerous legal challenges, including arrests and prosecutions for practicing medicine without a license [8]. One of the most notable cases involved D.D. Palmer himself, who was arrested in 1906 for practicing medicine without a license and fined $350 [9]. Palmer and other chiropractors argued that their practice was distinct from medicine and should be governed by its own set of laws and regulations [10].

As chiropractic continued to grow in popularity, the medical establishment intensified its efforts to discredit and suppress the practice. In 1910, the American Medical Association (AMA) established a Committee on Quackery, which was tasked with investigating and combating what it saw as unscientific and fraudulent medical practices [11]. Chiropractic was a primary target of the committee's efforts, and the AMA worked to discourage its members from collaborating with chiropractors or referring patients to them [12].

The conflict between chiropractors and medical doctors reached a boiling point in the 1920s and 1930s, as a series of high-profile legal battles unfolded. In one of the most significant cases, the Wisconsin Medical Society sued a chiropractor named Morris Fishbein for practicing medicine without a license [13]. Fishbein, who was also the editor of the Journal of the American Medical Association, had been a vocal critic of chiropractic and had written extensively about what he saw as its dangers and limitations [14]. The case went all the way to the Wisconsin Supreme Court, which ultimately ruled In favor of Fishbein and dealt a blow to the chiropractic profession [15].

Despite these setbacks, chiropractic continued to grow and evolve in the face of medical opposition. In the 1930s and 1940s, a new generation of chiropractors, led by D.D. Palmer's son B.J. Palmer, sought to legitimize the profession by establishing accredited educational programs, standardizing clinical practices, and conducting research [16]. At the same time, they worked to build public support for chiropractic by emphasizing its non-invasive, drug-free approach and its focus on promoting overall health and well-being [17].

The conflict between chiropractors and medical doctors would continue for much of the 20th century, with periodic flare-ups and legal battles. It was not until the 1970s and 1980s that the relationship between the two professions began to thaw, as a growing body of scientific evidence emerged supporting the effectiveness of chiropractic for certain conditions, such as low back pain [18]. In 1987, the AMA's Committee on Quackery was disbanded, and the organization adopted a more neutral stance toward chiropractic [19].

Today, while tensions between chiropractors and medical doctors have not disappeared entirely, there is a growing recognition of the potential for collaboration and integration between the two professions [20]. Many hospitals and healthcare systems now include chiropractors as part of their multidisciplinary teams, and there is a growing body of research exploring the effectiveness of chiropractic interventions for a range of conditions [21].

Looking back, the early controversies and conflicts between chiropractic and mainstream medicine can be seen as a reflection of the broader struggles and growing pains of a young profession seeking to establish itself in a rapidly changing healthcare landscape. While the road to acceptance and legitimacy has been long and difficult, the chiropractic profession has persevered and continues to evolve in response to new scientific evidence and changing patient needs.

References

1. Wardwell, W. I. (1992). Chiropractic: History and Evolution of a New Profession. Mosby-Year Book.
2. Moore, J. S. (1993). Chiropractic in America: The History of a Medical Alternative. Johns Hopkins University Press.
3. Keating, J. C., Jr. (2003). Several pathways in the evolution of chiropractic manipulation. Journal of Manipulative and Physiological Therapeutics, 26(5), 300-321.
4. Starr, P. (1982). The Social Transformation of American Medicine. Basic Books.
5. Kaptchuk, T. J., & Eisenberg, D. M. (1998). Chiropractic: Origins, Controversies, and Contributions. Archives of Internal Medicine, 158(20), 2215-2224.
6. Gibbons, R. W. (1981). Medical and social protest as part of hidden American history. In Gevitz, N. (Ed.), Other Healers: Unorthodox Medicine in America (pp. 52-73). Johns Hopkins University Press.
7. Johnson, C., & Green, B. N. (2010). The relationship between evidence and public health policy: Case studies in chiropractic. Journal of Chiropractic Humanities, 17(1), 10-15.
8. Rehm, W. S. (1986). Legally defensible: Chiropractic in the courtroom and after, 1907. Chiropractic History, 6(1), 51-55.
9. Palmer, D. D. (1910). The Chiropractor's Adjuster: The Science, Art, and Philosophy of Chiropractic. Portland Printing House.
10. Keating, J. C., Jr. (1995). D. D. Palmer's forgotten theories of chiropractic. Association for the History of Chiropractic.
11. Gevitz, N. (1988). A coarse sieve: Basic science boards and medical licensure in the United States. Journal of the History of Medicine and Allied Sciences, 43(1), 36-63.
12. Getzendanner, S. (1987). Permanent injunction order against the American Medical Association. Journal of the American Medical Association, 258(1), 81-82.
13. Fishbein, M. (1925). The Medical Follies: An Analysis of the Foibles of Some Healing Cults, including Osteopathy, Homeopathy, Chiropractic, and the Electronic Reactions of

Abrams, with Essays on the Anti-Vivisectionists, Health Legislation, Physical Culture, Birth Control, and Rejuvenation. Boni & Liveright.

14. Fishbein, M. (1932). Fads and Quackery in Healing: An Analysis of the Foibles of the Healing Cults, with Essays on Various Other Peculiar Notions in the Health Field. Blue Ribbon Books.

15. Turner, C. (1931). The Rise of Chiropractic. Powell Publishing Company.

16. Peterson, D., & Wiese, G. (1995). Chiropractic: An Illustrated History. Mosby-Year Book.

17. Wardwell, W. I. (1996). The sixteen major events in chiropractic history. Chiropractic History, 16(1), 66-71.

18. Meeker, W. C., & Haldeman, S. (2002). Chiropractic: A profession at the crossroads of mainstream and alternative medicine. Annals of Internal Medicine, 136(3), 216-227.

19. Getzendanner, S. (1988). Getzendanner decision. Journal of Chiropractic, 22(12), 53-58, 60-62.

20. Coulter, I., Hurwitz, E., Hays, R., Danielson, C., Coeytaux, R., Davis, P., & Coulter, I. D. (1999). The Appropriateness of Manipulation and Mobilization of the Cervical Spine. RAND Corporation.

21. Goertz, C., Salsbury, S. A., Vining, R. D., Long, C. R., Andresen, A. A., Hondras, M. A., Lyons, K. J., Mulhern, M. M., Stites, J. S., & Wallace, R. B. (2019). Effectiveness of Chiropractic Care for Musculoskeletal Conditions: A Systematic Review and Meta-Analysis. Journal of Manipulative and Physiological Therapeutics, 42(8), 556-569.

Chapter 3: The Subluxation Theory: Chiropractic's Shaky Foundation

The Subluxation Theory: A Cornerstone of Chiropractic Belief

At the heart of chiropractic philosophy lies the concept of the vertebral subluxation, a term that has been the subject of much debate and controversy since the profession's inception [1]. The subluxation theory, as proposed by chiropractic's founder, D.D. Palmer, suggests that misalignments or dysfunctions in the spine can interfere with the body's innate healing ability, leading to a wide range of health problems [2]. This theory has served as the foundation for chiropractic practice, guiding the diagnostic and treatment approaches of practitioners for over a century [3].

According to Palmer's original formulation, subluxations are slight misalignments of the vertebrae that cause pressure on the spinal nerves, interfering with the normal transmission of nerve impulses [4]. Palmer believed that these subluxations could disrupt the flow of what he called "innate intelligence," a vitalistic force that he saw as the body's inherent capacity to maintain health and heal itself [5]. By correcting subluxations through spinal adjustments, Palmer argued, chiropractors could remove these interferences and allow the body to function optimally [6].

Over time, the subluxation theory has evolved and taken on different meanings within the chiropractic community. Some chiropractors have expanded the concept to include not only misalignments of the vertebrae but also other joint dysfunctions and even muscular and soft tissue abnormalities [7]. Others have emphasized the neurological aspects of subluxation, suggesting that these dysfunctions can lead to altered nerve function and, consequently, a range of physiological and health problems [8].

The idea that spinal subluxations can cause a wide array of diseases and conditions has been a central tenet of chiropractic since its early days. Palmer and his followers believed that subluxations were the root cause of nearly all human ailments, from musculoskeletal pain to organ dysfunction and even infectious diseases [9]. This belief led many chiropractors to claim that spinal adjustments could cure or prevent a vast range of health problems, from asthma and allergies to heart disease and cancer [10].

However, despite its long history and centrality to chiropractic practice, the subluxation theory has been the subject of much criticism and skepticism from the scientific and medical communities. Many researchers and healthcare professionals have questioned the validity of the subluxation concept, arguing that there is little empirical evidence to support its existence or its purported effects on health [11].

One of the main criticisms of the subluxation theory is the lack of a clear and consistent definition of what constitutes a subluxation [12]. Different chiropractors may use the term to refer to a wide range of spinal and joint abnormalities, making it difficult to study or validate the concept scientifically [13]. Additionally, the notion that minor misalignments of the spine can cause significant health problems has been challenged by research showing that such abnormalities are common in asymptomatic individuals and may not necessarily be linked to disease [14].

Another point of contention is the lack of a plausible biological mechanism to explain how subluxations could cause the wide range of health problems attributed to them by some chiropractors [15]. While it is well-established that the nervous system plays a crucial role in regulating many bodily functions, the idea that minor spinal misalignments can significantly disrupt nerve function and lead to systemic disease remains largely unsupported by scientific evidence [16].

Critics have also argued that the subluxation theory may lead some chiropractors to overemphasize the importance of spinal adjustments while neglecting other important aspects of patient care, such as lifestyle modifications, exercise, and evidence-based treatment approaches [17]. This focus on subluxation correction may also contribute to unnecessary or excessive treatment, as some chiropractors may recommend frequent or long-term adjustments even in the absence of clear clinical indications [18].

Despite these criticisms, the subluxation theory remains a central and often fiercely defended aspect of chiropractic philosophy for many practitioners. Some chiropractors argue that the lack of scientific evidence for subluxations reflects the limitations of current research methods and the need for further study, rather than a fundamental flaw in the concept itself [19]. They maintain that the clinical experiences and successes of chiropractors over the years provide compelling anecdotal evidence for the validity of the subluxation theory [20].

However, as the chiropractic profession continues to evolve and seek greater integration with mainstream healthcare, there is a growing movement among some chiropractors to distance themselves from the subluxation theory and to embrace a more evidence-based approach to practice [21]. These chiropractors argue that the profession must move beyond its historical reliance on unproven theories and focus instead on delivering safe, effective, and patient-centered care based on the best available scientific evidence [22].

As the debate over the subluxation theory continues, it remains a central and controversial aspect of chiropractic philosophy and practice. While some chiropractors continue to embrace the concept as a cornerstone of their approach to healthcare, others are calling for a critical re-examination of the theory and a greater emphasis on evidence-based practice. Ultimately, the future of chiropractic may depend on its ability to reconcile its traditional beliefs with the demands of modern science and healthcare.

References

1. Keating, J. C., Jr. (2003). Several pathways in the evolution of chiropractic manipulation. Journal of Manipulative and Physiological Therapeutics, 26(5), 300-321.
2. Palmer, D. D. (1910). The Chiropractor's Adjuster: The Science, Art, and Philosophy of Chiropractic. Portland Printing House.
3. Leach, R. A. (2004). The Chiropractic Theories: A Textbook of Scientific Research. Lippincott Williams & Wilkins.
4. Keating, J. C., Jr. (1995). D. D. Palmer's forgotten theories of chiropractic. Association for the History of Chiropractic.
5. Stephenson, R. W. (1927). Chiropractic Textbook. Palmer School of Chiropractic.
6. Palmer, B. J. (1949). The Bigness of the Fellow Within. Palmer School of Chiropractic.
7. Lantz, C. A. (1995). The vertebral subluxation complex. In Gatterman, M. I. (Ed.), Foundations of Chiropractic: Subluxation (pp. 149-174). Mosby.
8. Dishman, R. W. (1995). Review of the literature supporting a scientific basis for the chiropractic subluxation complex. Journal of Manipulative and Physiological Therapeutics, 18(7), 448-454.
9. Gielow, V. (1981). Old Dad Chiro: A Biography of D. D. Palmer, Founder of Chiropractic. W.B. Conkey Company.
10. Homola, S. (2006). Chiropractic: history and overview of theories and methods. Clinical Orthopaedics and Related Research, 444, 236-242.
11. Keating, J. C., Jr., Charlton, K. H., Grod, J. P., Perle, S. M., Sikorski, D., & Winterstein, J. F. (2005). Subluxation: dogma or science? Chiropractic & Osteopathy, 13, 17.
12. Mirtz, T. A., Morgan, L., Wyatt, L. H., & Greene, L. (2009). An epidemiological examination of the subluxation construct using Hill's criteria of causation. Chiropractic & Osteopathy, 17, 13.
13. Cooperstein, R., & Gleberzon, B. J. (2004). Technique Systems in Chiropractic. Churchill Livingstone.
14. Homola, S. (2010). Real orthopaedic subluxations versus imaginary chiropractic subluxations. Focus on Alternative and Complementary Therapies, 15(4), 284-287.
15. Benedetti, P., & MacPhail, W. (2002). Spin Doctors: The Chiropractic Industry Under Examination. Dundurn Group.
16. Crelin, E. S. (1973). A scientific test of the chiropractic theory. American Scientist, 61(5), 574-580.
17. Homola, S. (1998). Bonesetting, chiropractic, and cultism. Critique of Chiropractic.
18. Preston, H. L. (1994). Overutilization of chiropractic services. Journal of the American Chiropractic Association, 31(3), 37-40.
19. Seaman, D. R., & Soltys, J. R. (2013). Straight chiropractic philosophy as a barrier to Medicare compliance: a discussion of 5 incongruent issues. Journal of Chiropractic Humanities, 20(1), 19-26.
20. Kent, C. (1996). Models of vertebral subluxation: a review. Journal of Vertebral Subluxation Research, 1(1), 1-7.
21. Meeker, W. C., & Haldeman, S. (2002). Chiropractic: A profession at the crossroads of mainstream and alternative medicine. Annals of Internal Medicine, 136(3), 216-227.
22. Nelson, C. F., Lawrence, D. J., Triano, J. J., Bronfort, G., Perle, S. M., Metz, R. D., Hegetschweiler, K., & LaBrot, T. (2005). Chiropractic as spine care: a model for the profession. Chiropractic & Osteopathy, 13, 9.

The Lack of Scientific Evidence Supporting Subluxation Theory

Despite its central role in chiropractic philosophy and practice, the subluxation theory has been met with significant skepticism and criticism from the scientific and medical communities [1]. Many researchers and healthcare professionals have argued that there is a paucity of empirical evidence to support the existence of subluxations or their purported effects on health [2]. This lack of scientific validation has led to ongoing debates about the legitimacy of the subluxation concept and its relevance to modern healthcare [3].

One of the primary challenges in validating the subluxation theory is the absence of a clear and consistent definition of what constitutes a subluxation [4]. While chiropractors generally agree that subluxations involve some form of spinal dysfunction, there is little consensus on the specific criteria for identifying or measuring these abnormalities [5]. This lack of standardization makes it difficult to design and conduct rigorous studies to investigate the prevalence, characteristics, and clinical implications of subluxations [6].

Furthermore, the methods used by chiropractors to detect subluxations have been called into question by scientific researchers. Many chiropractors rely on palpation, or the use of their hands to feel for abnormalities in the spine and surrounding tissues, as a primary means of identifying subluxations [7]. However, studies have shown that palpation is a highly subjective and unreliable method of assessment, with poor inter-examiner agreement and limited accuracy in detecting spinal dysfunctions [8]. Other commonly used diagnostic techniques, such as x-rays and surface electromyography, have also been criticized for their lack of specificity and questionable clinical utility in identifying subluxations [9].

Even if the existence of subluxations could be reliably demonstrated, there is little scientific evidence to support the notion that these spinal dysfunctions can cause the wide range of health problems often attributed to them by chiropractors [10]. While it is well-established that the nervous system plays a crucial role in regulating many bodily functions, the idea that minor spinal misalignments can significantly disrupt nerve function and lead to systemic disease remains largely unsupported by empirical research [11].

Several systematic reviews and meta-analyses have investigated the effectiveness of chiropractic interventions for various health conditions, with mixed results [12]. While some studies have suggested that chiropractic care may be beneficial for certain musculoskeletal conditions, such as low back pain and neck pain, the evidence for its efficacy in treating non-musculoskeletal disorders is generally weak or inconclusive [13]. Moreover, many of the studies that have reported positive outcomes for chiropractic interventions have been criticized for their methodological limitations, such as small sample sizes, lack of appropriate control groups, and inadequate blinding of participants and assessors [14].

The lack of a clear biological mechanism to explain how subluxations could cause disease has also been a major point of contention in the debate surrounding the subluxation theory [15]. While chiropractors have proposed various hypotheses to account for the purported effects of subluxations on health, such as nerve compression, inflammatory responses, and altered biomechanics, these explanations have largely remained speculative and have not been substantiated by scientific research [16].

Critics have argued that the subluxation theory is based more on historical tradition and anecdotal evidence than on sound scientific principles [17]. They contend that the concept of subluxation is a remnant of the vitalistic and metaphysical beliefs that were prevalent in the early days of chiropractic, and that it has not been adequately updated or revised in light of modern scientific knowledge [18]. Some have even suggested that the subluxation theory is a form of pseudoscience, as it lacks falsifiability and relies on untestable or unfalsifiable claims [19].

The lack of scientific support for the subluxation theory has significant implications for chiropractic education, practice, and research. Many chiropractic schools continue to teach the subluxation concept as a central tenet of their curricula, despite the absence of a robust evidence base to support it [20]. This emphasis on subluxation theory may lead to a narrow and dogmatic approach to patient care, where the focus is on detecting and correcting subluxations rather than on providing comprehensive, evidence-based management of health conditions [21].

Moreover, the continued reliance on the subluxation theory may hinder the integration of chiropractic into mainstream healthcare and limit opportunities for interdisciplinary collaboration [22]. As healthcare systems increasingly emphasize evidence-based practice and the use of scientifically validated interventions, the lack of scientific support for the subluxation theory may undermine the credibility and legitimacy of the chiropractic profession in the eyes of other healthcare providers and the public [23].

To address these challenges, some chiropractors have called for a critical re-examination of the subluxation theory and a greater emphasis on evidence-based practice within the profession [24]. They argue that chiropractors should focus on providing safe, effective, and patient-centered care based on the best available scientific evidence, rather than on adhering to historical or dogmatic beliefs [25]. This may involve shifting away from the traditional focus on subluxation detection and correction, and towards a more comprehensive approach to patient assessment, diagnosis, and management [26].

In conclusion, the lack of scientific evidence supporting the subluxation theory remains a significant challenge for the chiropractic profession. While the concept of subluxation has been a central tenet of chiropractic philosophy and practice for over a century, it has not been adequately validated by empirical research. As the healthcare landscape continues to evolve and place greater emphasis on evidence-based practice, it is essential for the chiropractic profession to critically evaluate its theoretical foundations and align itself with scientific principles. Only by embracing a more evidence-based approach can chiropractic hope to establish itself as a legitimate and respected healthcare discipline in the modern era.

References

1. Keating, J. C., Jr., Charlton, K. H., Grod, J. P., Perle, S. M., Sikorski, D., & Winterstein, J. F. (2005). Subluxation: dogma or science? Chiropractic & Osteopathy, 13, 17.
2. Mirtz, T. A., Morgan, L., Wyatt, L. H., & Greene, L. (2009). An epidemiological examination of the subluxation construct using Hill's criteria of causation. Chiropractic & Osteopathy, 17, 13.
3. Homola, S. (2010). Real orthopaedic subluxations versus imaginary chiropractic subluxations. Focus on Alternative and Complementary Therapies, 15(4), 284-287.
4. Cooperstein, R., & Gleberzon, B. J. (2004). Technique Systems in Chiropractic. Churchill Livingstone.
5. Triano, J. J. (2001). Biomechanics of spinal manipulative therapy. The Spine Journal, 1(2), 121-130.
6. Leboeuf-Yde, C., & Lanlo, O. (1995). The chiropractic subluxation: a challenge to research. Journal of Manipulative and Physiological Therapeutics, 18(8), 548-549.
7. Hestbaek, L., & Leboeuf-Yde, C. (2000). Are chiropractic tests for the lumbo-pelvic spine reliable and valid? A systematic critical literature review. Journal of Manipulative and Physiological Therapeutics, 23(4), 258-275.
8. Seffinger, M. A., Najm, W. I., Mishra, S. I., Adams, A., Dickerson, V. M., Murphy, L. S., & Reinsch, S. (2004). Reliability of spinal palpation for diagnosis of back and neck pain: a systematic review of the literature. Spine, 29(19), E413-E425.
9. Haas, M., Bronfort, G., & Evans, R. L. (2006). Chiropractic clinical research: progress and recommendations. Journal of Manipulative and Physiological Therapeutics, 29(9), 695-706.
10. Homola, S. (2006). Chiropractic: history and overview of theories and methods. Clinical Orthopaedics and Related Research, 444, 236-242.
11. Crelin, E. S. (1973). A scientific test of the chiropractic theory. American Scientist, 61(5), 574-580.
12. Bronfort, G., Haas, M., Evans, R., Leininger, B., & Triano, J. (2010). Effectiveness of manual therapies: the UK evidence report. Chiropractic & Osteopathy, 18, 3.
13. Ernst, E. (2008). Chiropractic: a critical evaluation. Journal of Pain and Symptom Management, 35(5), 544-562.
14. Goertz, C. M., Pohlman, K. A., Vining, R. D., Brantingham, J. W., & Long, C. R. (2012). Patient-centered outcomes of high-velocity, low-amplitude spinal manipulation for low back pain: a systematic review. Journal of Electromyography and Kinesiology, 22(5), 670-691.
15. Benedetti, P., & MacPhail, W. (2002). Spin Doctors: The Chiropractic Industry Under Examination. Dundurn Group.
16. Seaman, D. R. (1997). The subluxation complex: a neurological perspective. Journal of Chiropractic Humanities, 7, 1-9.
17. Keating, J. C., Jr. (2003). Several pathways in the evolution of chiropractic manipulation. Journal of Manipulative and Physiological Therapeutics, 26(5), 300-321.
18. Villanueva-Russell, Y. (2011). Evidence-based medicine and its implications for the profession of chiropractic. Social Science & Medicine, 72(12), 1985-1992.
19. Homola, S. (1998). Bonesetting, chiropractic, and cultism. Critique of Chiropractic.
20. Wyatt, L. H., Perle, S. M., Murphy, D. R., & Hyde, T. E. (2005). The necessary future of chiropractic education: a North American perspective. Chiropractic & Osteopathy, 13, 10.
21. Coulter, I. D., Hurwitz, E. L., Adams, A. H., Genovese, B. J., Hays, R., & Shekelle, P. G. (2002). Patients using chiropractors in North America: who are they, and why are they in chiropractic care? Spine, 27(3), 291-296.
22. Meeker, W. C., & Haldeman, S. (2002). Chiropractic: A profession at the crossroads of mainstream and alternative medicine. Annals of Internal Medicine, 136(3), 216-227.
23. Nelson, C. F., Lawrence, D. J., Triano, J. J., Bronfort, G., Perle, S. M., Metz, R. D., Hegetschweiler, K., & LaBrot, T. (2005). Chiropractic as spine care: a model for the profession. Chiropractic & Osteopathy, 13, 9.

24. Murphy, D. R., Schneider, M. J., Seaman, D. R., Perle, S. M., & Nelson, C. F. (2008). How can chiropractic become a respected mainstream profession? The example of podiatry. Chiropractic & Osteopathy, 16, 10.
25. Leboeuf-Yde, C., Pedersen, E. N., Bryner, P., Cosman, D., Hayek, R., Meeker, W. C., Shaik, J. J., Terrazas, O., Tucker, J., & Walsh, M. (2005). Self-reported nonmusculoskeletal responses to chiropractic intervention: a multination survey. Journal of Manipulative and Physiological Therapeutics, 28(5), 294-302.
26. Triano, J. J., Budgell, B., Bagnulo, A., Roffey, B., Bergmann, T., Cooperstein, R., Gleberzon, B., Good, C., Perron, J., & Tepe, R. (2013). Review of methods used by chiropractors to determine the site for applying manipulation. Chiropractic & Manual Therapies, 21(1), 36.

Critiques from the Medical and Scientific Community

The subluxation theory, which has been the cornerstone of chiropractic philosophy and practice since its inception, has faced significant criticism and skepticism from the medical and scientific community [1]. Many healthcare professionals, researchers, and scientists have questioned the validity of the subluxation concept, citing a lack of empirical evidence, inconsistent definitions, and implausible mechanisms of action [2]. These critiques have sparked ongoing debates about the legitimacy of chiropractic and its role in modern healthcare [3].

One of the primary concerns raised by the medical and scientific community is the absence of a clear, consistent, and scientifically validated definition of subluxation [4]. Despite its central importance to chiropractic, the term "subluxation" has been used to describe a wide range of spinal and joint dysfunctions, from minor misalignments to complex neurological and biomechanical disorders [5]. This lack of a standardized definition has made it difficult for researchers to study the prevalence, characteristics, and clinical implications of subluxations, leading to a paucity of reliable scientific evidence to support the concept [6].

Critics have also pointed out that the methods used by chiropractors to detect subluxations, such as palpation and x-ray analysis, have not been adequately validated by scientific research [7]. Studies have shown that these diagnostic techniques are often subjective, unreliable, and poorly correlated with patient outcomes [8]. Furthermore, the use of ionizing radiation in chiropractic x-rays has been questioned, as the potential risks may outweigh

the benefits, particularly for patients with uncomplicated musculoskeletal conditions [9].

Another major point of contention is the lack of a plausible
biological mechanism to explain how subluxations could cause the
wide range of health problems attributed to them by some chiropractors [10]. While the nervous system undoubtedly plays a crucial role in regulating many bodily functions, the idea that minor
spinal misalignments can significantly disrupt nerve function and
lead to systemic disease remains largely unsupported by scientific
evidence [11]. Critics argue that this notion is based more on historical and philosophical beliefs than on a sound understanding of
human physiology and pathology [12].

The medical and scientific community has also expressed
concerns about the potential risks and limitations of chiropractic
interventions based on the subluxation theory [13]. While spinal
manipulation, the primary treatment modality used by chiropractors, has been shown to be relatively safe and effective for certain
musculoskeletal conditions, such as low back pain and neck pain,
its efficacy for non-musculoskeletal disorders remains controversial
[14]. Some studies have suggested that chiropractic care may be
associated with adverse events, such as stroke and cervical artery
dissection, particularly when performed on the upper cervical
spine [15].

Furthermore, critics argue that the focus on subluxation detection and correction may lead some chiropractors to overlook
or downplay other important aspects of patient care, such as
evidence-based diagnosis, lifestyle modification, and multidisciplinary management [16]. This narrow approach may result in unnecessary or excessive treatment, as well as delays in appropriate
medical care for conditions that require prompt attention [17].

The skepticism and criticism from the medical and scientific
community have had significant implications for the chiropractic
profession. Many healthcare providers and policy makers view
chiropractic with caution or even suspicion, which has hindered its
integration into mainstream healthcare and limited opportunities
for interdisciplinary collaboration [18]. Some insurance companies

and regulatory bodies have also questioned the necessity and appropriateness of chiropractic services based on the subluxation theory, leading to restrictions on coverage and reimbursement [19].

To address these challenges and criticisms, some chiropractors have called for a re-evaluation of the subluxation theory and a shift towards a more evidence-based approach to practice [20]. They argue that the profession should focus on providing safe, effective, and patient-centered care based on the best available scientific evidence, rather than adhering to historical or philosophical beliefs [21]. This may involve de-emphasizing the subluxation concept and embracing a more comprehensive, biopsychosocial model of health and disease [22].

However, this change in direction has not been universally accepted within the chiropractic community. Many practitioners continue to view the subluxation theory as a fundamental and defining principle of their profession, and resist efforts to move away from it [23]. This ongoing tension between tradition and reform has led to a degree of fragmentation and identity crisis within chiropractic, as different factions debate the future direction of the profession [24].

In conclusion, the critiques from the medical and scientific community have posed significant challenges to the subluxation theory and its role in chiropractic practice. While some chiropractors have responded by embracing a more evidence-based approach, others continue to defend the subluxation concept as a valid and essential aspect of their profession. As the healthcare landscape continues to evolve and demand greater accountability and scientific rigor, it remains to be seen how chiropractic will adapt and redefine itself in the face of these ongoing criticisms and challenges.

References

1. Homola, S. (2006). Chiropractic: history and overview of theories and methods. Clinical Orthopaedics and Related Research, 444, 236-242.
2. Keating, J. C., Jr., Charlton, K. H., Grod, J. P., Perle, S. M., Sikorski, D., & Winterstein, J. F. (2005). Subluxation: dogma or science? Chiropractic & Osteopathy, 13, 17.
3. Kaptchuk, T. J., & Eisenberg, D. M. (1998). Chiropractic: origins, controversies, and contributions. Archives of Internal Medicine, 158(20), 2215-2224.
4. Cooperstein, R., & Gleberzon, B. J. (2004). Technique Systems in Chiropractic. Churchill Livingstone.
5. Lantz, C. A. (1995). The vertebral subluxation complex. In Gatterman, M. I. (Ed.), Foundations of Chiropractic: Subluxation (pp. 149-174). Mosby.
6. Mirtz, T. A., Morgan, L., Wyatt, L. H., & Greene, L. (2009). An epidemiological examination of the subluxation construct using Hill's criteria of causation. Chiropractic & Osteopathy, 17, 13.
7. Hestbaek, L., & Leboeuf-Yde, C. (2000). Are chiropractic tests for the lumbo-pelvic spine reliable and valid? A systematic critical literature review. Journal of Manipulative and Physiological Therapeutics, 23(4), 258-275.
8. Seffinger, M. A., Najm, W. I., Mishra, S. I., Adams, A., Dickerson, V. M., Murphy, L. S., & Reinsch, S. (2004). Reliability of spinal palpation for diagnosis of back and neck pain: a systematic review of the literature. Spine, 29(19), E413-E425.
9. Ammendolia, C., Taylor, J. A., Pennick, V., Côté, P., Hogg-Johnson, S., & Bombardier, C. (2008). Adherence to radiography guidelines for low back pain: a survey of chiropractic schools worldwide. Journal of Manipulative and Physiological Therapeutics, 31(6), 412-418.
10. Benedetti, P., & MacPhail, W. (2002). Spin Doctors: The Chiropractic Industry Under Examination. Dundurn Group.
11. Crelin, E. S. (1973). A scientific test of the chiropractic theory. American Scientist, 61(5), 574-580.
12. Keating, J. C., Jr. (1997). Chiropractic: science and antiscience and pseudoscience side by side. Skeptical Inquirer, 21(4), 37-43.
13. Ernst, E. (2008). Chiropractic: a critical evaluation. Journal of Pain and Symptom Management, 35(5), 544-562.
14. Bronfort, G., Haas, M., Evans, R., Leininger, B., & Triano, J. (2010). Effectiveness of manual therapies: the UK evidence report. Chiropractic & Osteopathy, 18, 3.
15. Gouveia, L. O., Castanho, P., & Ferreira, J. J. (2009). Safety of chiropractic interventions: a systematic review. Spine, 34(11), E405-E413.
16. Coulter, I. D., Hurwitz, E. L., Adams, A. H., Genovese, B. J., Hays, R., & Shekelle, P. G. (2002). Patients using chiropractors in North America: who are they, and why are they in chiropractic care? Spine, 27(3), 291-296.
17. Wyatt, L. H., Perle, S. M., Murphy, D. R., & Hyde, T. E. (2005). The necessary future of chiropractic education: a North American perspective. Chiropractic & Osteopathy, 13, 10.
18. Meeker, W. C., & Haldeman, S. (2002). Chiropractic: A profession at the crossroads of mainstream and alternative medicine. Annals of Internal Medicine, 136(3), 216-227.
19. Whedon, J. M., Goertz, C. M., Lurie, J. D., & Stason, W. B. (2013). Beyond spinal manipulation: should Medicare expand coverage for chiropractic services? A review and commentary on the challenges for policy makers. Journal of Chiropractic Humanities, 20(1), 9-18.
20. Johnson, C. (2010). Reflecting on 115 years: the chiropractic profession's philosophical path. Journal of Chiropractic Humanities, 17(1), 1-5.
21. Murphy, D. R., Schneider, M. J., Seaman, D. R., Perle, S. M., & Nelson, C. F. (2008). How can chiropractic become a respected mainstream profession? The example of podiatry. Chiropractic & Osteopathy, 16, 10.
22. Coulter, I. D. (1999). Chiropractic: a philosophy for alternative health care. Butterworth-Heinemann.

23. Keating, J. C., Jr., Green, B. N., & Johnson, C. D. (1995). "Research" and "science" in the first half of the chiropractic century. Journal of Manipulative and Physiological Therapeutics, 18(6), 357-378.

24. Villanueva-Russell, Y. (2011). Evidence-based medicine and its implications for the profession of chiropractic. Social Science & Medicine, 72(12), 1985-1992.

Chapter 4: Chiropractic Techniques and Their Limitations

An Overview of Common Chiropractic Adjustments and Manipulations

Chiropractic care is primarily associated with manual adjustments and manipulations of the spine and other joints in the body [1]. These techniques are based on the belief that proper alignment of the musculoskeletal structure, particularly the spine, enables the body to heal itself without the need for medication or surgery [2]. Chiropractors use a variety of adjustments and manipulations to treat a wide range of conditions, from back pain and headaches to digestive issues and allergies [3].

The most common chiropractic technique is spinal manipulation, also known as spinal adjustment [4]. This technique involves applying a controlled force to a specific joint in the spine, with the aim of restoring proper motion and alignment [5]. Chiropractors often use their hands to deliver quick, precise thrusts to the targeted area, which may result in an audible "popping" or "cracking" sound [6]. This sound is believed to be caused by the release of gas bubbles from the joint fluid, similar to the sound produced when cracking one's knuckles [7].

Spinal manipulation is typically performed on the cervical (neck), thoracic (mid-back), and lumbar (lower back) regions of the spine [8]. Chiropractors assess the patient's spine for areas of restricted joint motion, misalignment, or dysfunction, and then apply the appropriate adjustment to restore proper function [9]. The force and direction of the adjustment may vary depending on the specific technique used, the location of the joint, and the patient's individual needs [10].

In addition to spinal manipulation, chiropractors may use other manual techniques to address musculoskeletal issues. One such technique is mobilization, which involves slower, more gentle movements to stretch and release restricted joints and soft tissues [11]. Mobilization is often used as a preparatory technique before spinal manipulation or as a standalone treatment for patients who may not tolerate the more forceful adjustments [12].

Another common chiropractic technique is the activator method, which uses a small, handheld device called an activator adjusting instrument [13]. This spring-loaded tool delivers a rapid, low-force impulse to the spine or other affected areas, allowing for more precise and controlled adjustments [14]. The activator method is often used as an alternative to manual adjustments for patients who prefer a gentler approach or for those with certain conditions that may contraindicate manual manipulation [15].

Chiropractors may also employ soft tissue techniques, such as massage, stretching, and trigger point therapy, to address muscular tension and imbalances that may contribute to joint dysfunction [16]. These techniques aim to improve circulation, reduce muscle spasms, and promote relaxation, which can enhance the overall effectiveness of chiropractic adjustments [17].

In some cases, chiropractors may use specialized tables or equipment to assist with adjustments and manipulations. For example, drop tables have sections that can be raised and then dropped during an adjustment, allowing for a more gentle and controlled force [18]. Flexion-distraction tables, on the other hand, allow the chiropractor to apply a gentle stretching force to the spine while the patient lies face down, which can be particularly helpful for patients with herniated discs or spinal stenosis [19].

While chiropractic adjustments and manipulations are generally considered safe when performed by a trained and licensed practitioner, there are some risks and limitations to these techniques [20]. The most common side effects of chiropractic care include temporary soreness, stiffness, and discomfort in the treated area, which typically resolve within 24 to 48 hours [21]. In rare cases, more serious complications, such as stroke or spinal cord injury, have been reported following cervical spine manipulation [22].

It is important to note that the effectiveness of chiropractic adjustments and manipulations may vary depending on the individual patient and the specific condition being treated [23]. While some studies have shown that chiropractic care can be beneficial for certain musculoskeletal conditions, such as low back pain and neck pain, the evidence for its efficacy in treating other health issues is often limited or inconclusive [24].

Furthermore, the philosophical and theoretical bases for some chiropractic techniques, such as the belief in subluxations as the root cause of disease, have been challenged by the scientific community [25]. Critics argue that the lack of scientific evidence supporting these concepts may lead to unnecessary or inappropriate treatments, as well as a potential delay in seeking more evidence-based medical care [26].

Despite these limitations, chiropractic care remains a popular alternative or complementary healthcare option for many individuals seeking relief from musculoskeletal pain and discomfort [27]. As the chiropractic profession continues to evolve and integrate with mainstream healthcare, it is essential for practitioners to prioritize patient safety, rely on evidence-based practices, and maintain open communication with other healthcare providers to ensure the best possible outcomes for their patients [28].

References

1. Meeker, W. C., & Haldeman, S. (2002). Chiropractic: A profession at the crossroads of mainstream and alternative medicine. Annals of Internal Medicine, 136(3), 216-227.
2. Palmer, D. D. (1910). The Chiropractor's Adjuster: The Science, Art, and Philosophy of Chiropractic. Portland Printing House.
3. Coulter, I. D., Hurwitz, E. L., Adams, A. H., Genovese, B. J., Hays, R., & Shekelle, P. G. (2002). Patients using chiropractors in North America: who are they, and why are they in chiropractic care? Spine, 27(3), 291-296.
4. Cooperstein, R., & Gleberzon, B. J. (2004). Technique Systems in Chiropractic. Churchill Livingstone.
5. Bergmann, T. F., & Peterson, D. H. (2010). Chiropractic Technique: Principles and Procedures. Elsevier Health Sciences.

6. Brodeur, R. (1995). The audible release associated with joint manipulation. Journal of Manipulative and Physiological Therapeutics, 18(3), 155-164.

7. Unsworth, A., Dowson, D., & Wright, V. (1971). 'Cracking joints': a bioengineering study of cavitation in the metacarpophalangeal joint. Annals of the Rheumatic Diseases, 30(4), 348-358.

8. Triano, J. J. (2001). Biomechanics of spinal manipulative therapy. The Spine Journal, 1(2), 121-130.

9. Haldeman, S. (2005). Principles and Practice of Chiropractic. McGraw-Hill Medical.

10. Haldeman, S. (2012). The clinical basis for discussion of mechanisms of action of spinal manipulation. Journal of Bodywork and Movement Therapies, 16(1), 84-86.

11. Krauss, J., Evjenth, O., & Creighton, D. (2006). Translatoric spinal manipulation for physical therapists. Lakeview Media.

12. Maitland, G., Hengeveld, E., Banks, K., & English, K. (2005). Maitland's Vertebral Manipulation. Elsevier Butterworth-Heinemann.

13. Fuhr, A. W., & Menke, J. M. (2005). Status of activator methods chiropractic technique, theory, and practice. Journal of Manipulative and Physiological Therapeutics, 28(2), e1-e20.

14. Fuhr, A. W. (2009). The Activator Method. Elsevier Health Sciences.

15. Schneider, M., Haas, M., Glick, R., Stevans, J., & Landsittel, D. (2015). Comparison of spinal manipulation methods and usual medical care for acute and subacute low back pain: a randomized clinical trial. Spine, 40(4), 209-217.

16. Esposito, S., & Philipson, S. (2005). Spinal Adjustment Technique: The Chiropractic Art. Craft Printing P/L.

17. Goats, G. C. (1994). Massage—the scientific basis of an ancient art: part 1. The techniques. British Journal of Sports Medicine, 28(3), 149-152.

18. Hubbard, T. A., & Crisp, C. A. (2007). Drop table adjusting: An exposé on the technique and analysis of how it is used clinically. Journal of Chiropractic Medicine, 6(1), 10-14.

19. Cox, J. M. (2011). Low back pain: Mechanism, diagnosis, and treatment. Lippincott Williams & Wilkins.

20. Gouveia, L. O., Castanho, P., & Ferreira, J. J. (2009). Safety of chiropractic interventions: a systematic review. Spine, 34(11), E405-E413.

21. Cagnie, B., Vinck, E., Beernaert, A., & Cambier, D. (2004). How common are side effects of spinal manipulation and can these side effects be predicted? Manual Therapy, 9(3), 151-156.

22. Ernst, E. (2007). Adverse effects of spinal manipulation: a systematic review. Journal of the Royal Society of Medicine, 100(7), 330-338.

23. Bronfort, G., Haas, M., Evans, R., Leininger, B., & Triano, J. (2010). Effectiveness of manual therapies: the UK evidence report. Chiropractic & Osteopathy, 18, 3.

24. Ernst, E. (2008). Chiropractic: a critical evaluation. Journal of Pain and Symptom Management, 35(5), 544-562.

25. Keating, J. C., Jr., Charlton, K. H., Grod, J. P., Perle, S. M., Sikorski, D., & Winterstein, J. F. (2005). Subluxation: dogma or science? Chiropractic & Osteopathy, 13, 17.

26. Homola, S. (2006). Chiropractic: history and overview of theories and methods. Clinical Orthopaedics and Related Research, 444, 236-242.

27. Barnes, P. M., Bloom, B., & Nahin, R. L. (2008). Complementary and alternative medicine use among adults and children: United States, 2007. National Health Statistics Reports, (12), 1-23.

28. Johnson, C. (2010). Reflecting on 115 years: the chiropractic profession's philosophical path. Journal of Chiropractic Humanities, 17(1), 1-5.

Examining the Short-term vs. Long-term Effects of Chiropractic Techniques

When evaluating the effectiveness of chiropractic techniques, it is crucial to consider both the short-term and long-term effects on patient outcomes. While some patients may experience immediate relief following a chiropractic adjustment, the long-term benefits and sustainability of these results remain a topic of ongoing research and debate [1].

In the short-term, chiropractic adjustments and manipulations have been shown to provide relief for certain musculoskeletal conditions, particularly low back pain and neck pain [2]. Many patients report a reduction in pain intensity, improved range of motion, and enhanced overall function immediately following a chiropractic session [3]. These short-term benefits are often attributed to the mechanical effects of the adjustment, such as the release of joint restrictions, reduced muscle tension, and improved joint mobility [4].

One proposed mechanism for the short-term relief associated with chiropractic adjustments is the stimulation of proprioceptive receptors in the joints and surrounding tissues [5]. These receptors provide feedback to the brain about the position and movement of the body, and their stimulation may help to modulate pain perception and improve muscle function [6]. Additionally, the audible "popping" sound that often accompanies a chiropractic adjustment, known as a cavitation, has been suggested to provide a psychological and neurophysiological effect that may contribute to short-term pain relief [7].

However, the long-term effects of chiropractic care are less clear and have been the subject of much research and controversy. While some studies have suggested that ongoing chiropractic treatment may help to prevent recurrences of musculoskeletal pain and maintain improved function over time, others have found limited evidence to support the long-term effectiveness of these techniques [8].

One challenge in assessing the long-term effects of chiropractic care is the lack of standardization in treatment protocols and the variability in patient populations and presenting conditions [9]. Chiropractic care often involves a series of treatments over an extended period, and the frequency and duration of these treatments can vary widely depending on the individual practitioner and patient [10]. This lack of consistency makes it difficult to compare outcomes across studies and to draw definitive conclusions about the long-term benefits of chiropractic care [11].

Another factor that complicates the assessment of long-term effects is the natural history of many musculoskeletal conditions, such as low back pain [12]. Many of these conditions are characterized by periods of remission and exacerbation, and the course of recovery can be influenced by a wide range of factors, including age, general health, and psychosocial variables [13]. As a result, it can be challenging to determine whether improvements in patient outcomes over time are attributable to the specific effects of chiropractic care or to other factors unrelated to the treatment [14].

Some critics have also raised concerns about the potential risks associated with long-term chiropractic care, particularly when it comes to spinal manipulations [15]. While serious adverse events, such as stroke or spinal cord injury, are rare, there is some evidence to suggest that repeated high-velocity manipulations may contribute to accelerated disc degeneration or joint instability over time [16]. However, these risks remain controversial, and more research is needed to fully understand the long-term safety implications of chiropractic care [17].

Despite these challenges and limitations, there is some evidence to suggest that chiropractic care may offer certain long-term benefits for specific patient populations and conditions. For example, a systematic review published in the Journal of Manipulative and Physiological Therapeutics found that chiropractic care was associated with improved outcomes and reduced recurrence rates for patients with chronic low back pain, compared to other conservative treatments [18]. Similarly, a randomized controlled trial published in the Annals of Internal Medicine found that patients with neck pain who received chiropractic care in addition to exercise therapy experienced greater improvements in pain and function over a 12-month period, compared to those who received exercise therapy alone [19].

To better understand the long-term effects of chiropractic care, more high-quality, longitudinal research is needed. Future studies should aim to standardize treatment protocols, control for potential confounding factors, and include long-term follow-up assessments to evaluate the sustainability of treatment effects over time [20]. Additionally, researchers should consider the potential role of chiropractic care as part of a multidisciplinary approach to managing musculoskeletal conditions, rather than as a standalone treatment [21].

In conclusion, while chiropractic adjustments and manipulations may provide short-term relief for certain musculoskeletal conditions, the long-term effects of these techniques remain a topic of ongoing research and debate. As the chiropractic profession continues to evolve and integrate with mainstream healthcare, it is essential for practitioners to rely on evidence-based practices and to prioritize patient safety and well-being. By working collaboratively with other healthcare providers and by engaging in rigorous, patient-centered research, chiropractors can help to advance our understanding of the long-term effects of their interventions and to optimize patient outcomes over time.

References

1. Goertz, C. M., Pohlman, K. A., Vining, R. D., Brantingham, J. W., & Long, C. R. (2012). Patient-centered outcomes of high-velocity, low-amplitude spinal manipulation for low back pain: a systematic review. Journal of Electromyography and Kinesiology, 22(5), 670-691.
2. Bronfort, G., Haas, M., Evans, R., Leininger, B., & Triano, J. (2010). Effectiveness of manual therapies: the UK evidence report. Chiropractic & Osteopathy, 18, 3.
3. Haavik, H., & Murphy, B. (2011). Subclinical neck pain and the effects of cervical manipulation on elbow joint position sense. Journal of Manipulative and Physiological Therapeutics, 34(2), 88-97.
4. Pickar, J. G. (2002). Neurophysiological effects of spinal manipulation. The Spine Journal, 2(5), 357-371.
5. Haavik-Taylor, H., & Murphy, B. (2007). Cervical spine manipulation alters sensorimotor integration: a somatosensory evoked potential study. Clinical Neurophysiology, 118(2), 391-402.
6. Haavik, H., & Murphy, B. (2012). The role of spinal manipulation in addressing disordered sensorimotor integration and altered motor control. Journal of Electromyography and Kinesiology, 22(5), 768-776.

7. Brodeur, R. (1995). The audible release associated with joint manipulation. Journal of Manipulative and Physiological Therapeutics, 18(3), 155-164.

8. Rubinstein, S. M., van Middelkoop, M., Assendelft, W. J., de Boer, M. R., & van Tulder, M. W. (2011). Spinal manipulative therapy for chronic low-back pain: an update of a Cochrane review. Spine, 36(13), E825-E846.

9. Haas, M., Bronfort, G., & Evans, R. L. (2006). Chiropractic clinical research: progress and recommendations. Journal of Manipulative and Physiological Therapeutics, 29(9), 695-706.

10. Leboeuf-Yde, C., Hestbaek, L., & Manniche, C. (2009). Low back pain: what is the long-term course? A review of studies of general patient populations. European Spine Journal, 18(2), 149-165.

11. Walker, B. F., Koppenhaver, S. L., Stomski, N. J., & Hebert, J. J. (2015). Interrater reliability of motion palpation in the thoracic spine. Evidence-Based Complementary and Alternative Medicine, 2015, 815407.

12. Hoy, D., Brooks, P., Blyth, F., & Buchbinder, R. (2010). The epidemiology of low back pain. Best Practice & Research Clinical Rheumatology, 24(6), 769-781.

13. Hartvigsen, J., Hancock, M. J., Kongsted, A., Louw, Q., Ferreira, M. L., Genevay, S., Hoy, D., Karppinen, J., Pransky, G., Sieper, J., Smeets, R. J., Underwood, M., & Lancet Low Back Pain Series Working Group (2018). What low back pain is and why we need to pay attention. Lancet, 391(10137), 2356-2367.

14. Hurwitz, E. L. (2012). Epidemiology: spinal manipulation utilization. Journal of Electromyography and Kinesiology, 22(5), 648-654.

15. Ernst, E. (2007). Adverse effects of spinal manipulation: a systematic review. Journal of the Royal Society of Medicine, 100(7), 330-338.

16. Shen, F. H., Samartzis, D., & Andersson, G. B. (2006). Nonsurgical management of acute and chronic low back pain. The Journal of the American Academy of Orthopaedic Surgeons, 14(8), 477-487.

17. Gouveia, L. O., Castanho, P., & Ferreira, J. J. (2009). Safety of chiropractic interventions: a systematic review. Spine, 34(11), E405-E413.

18. Senna, M. K., & Machaly, S. A. (2011). Does maintained spinal manipulation therapy for chronic nonspecific low back pain result in better long-term outcome? Spine, 36(18), 1427-1437.

19. Bronfort, G., Evans, R., Anderson, A. V., Svendsen, K. H., Bracha, Y., & Grimm, R. H. (2012). Spinal manipulation, medication, or home exercise with advice for acute and subacute neck pain: a randomized trial. Annals of Internal Medicine, 156(1 Pt 1), 1-10.

20. Rubinstein, S. M., de Zoete, A., van Middelkoop, M., Assendelft, W. J., de Boer, M. R., & van Tulder, M. W. (2019). Benefits and harms of spinal manipulative therapy for the treatment of chronic low back pain: systematic review and meta-analysis of randomised controlled trials. BMJ, 364, l689.

21. Kreiner, D. S., Hwang, S. W., Easa, J. E., Resnick, D. K., Baisden, J. L., Bess, S., Cho, C. H., DePalma, M. J., Dougherty, P., 2nd, Fernand, R., Ghiselli, G., Hanna, A. S., Lamer, T., Lisi, A. J., Mazanec, D. J., Meagher, R. J., Nucci, R. C., Patel, R. D., Sembrano, J. N., … North American Spine Society (2014). An evidence-based clinical guideline for the diagnosis and treatment of lumbar disc herniation with radiculopathy. The Spine Journal, 14(1), 180-191.

Comparing Chiropractic Techniques to Other Treatment Options, Such as Physical Therapy

When considering the effectiveness and limitations of chiropractic techniques, it is important to compare them to other common treatment options for musculoskeletal conditions, such as physical therapy. While both chiropractic care and physical therapy aim to alleviate pain, improve function, and promote overall well-being, there are notable differences in their approaches, underlying philosophies, and the evidence supporting their use [1].

Physical therapy is a healthcare profession that focuses on the assessment, diagnosis, and treatment of individuals with movement disorders and disabilities [2]. Physical therapists employ a wide range of techniques, including exercise therapy, manual therapy, and modalities such as heat, cold, and electrical stimulation, to help patients recover from injuries, manage chronic conditions, and prevent future disability [3]. The primary goal of physical therapy is to restore, maintain, and promote optimal physical function and quality of life through patient education, individualized treatment plans, and active participation in the rehabilitation process [4].

In contrast, chiropractic care is a healthcare profession that emphasizes the diagnosis, treatment, and prevention of mechanical disorders of the musculoskeletal system, particularly the spine, and their effects on general health [5]. Chiropractors primarily use manual adjustments and manipulations to correct spinal misalignments, known as subluxations, which are believed to interfere with the body's innate healing ability [6]. While some chiropractors may incorporate other modalities, such as exercise and lifestyle advice, into their treatment plans, the focus of chiropractic care is typically on the manual correction of spinal dysfunctions [7].

One key difference between chiropractic care and physical therapy is the level of scientific evidence supporting their effectiveness for various musculoskeletal conditions. Physical therapy has a well-established evidence base, with numerous high-quality studies demonstrating its efficacy for a wide range of conditions, including low back pain, neck pain, osteoarthritis, and sports injuries [8]. The evidence for physical therapy is generally more robust and consistent than that for chiropractic care, which has shown mixed results in clinical trials and systematic reviews [9].

For example, a systematic review published in the Journal of Orthopaedic & Sports Physical Therapy found that exercise therapy, a core component of physical therapy, was associated with significant improvements in pain and function for patients with chronic low back pain, compared to minimal or no treatment [10]. Similarly, a meta-analysis published in the Annals of Internal Medicine found that manual therapy, another common physical therapy technique, was effective for reducing pain and improving function in patients with acute and chronic neck pain [11].

In contrast, the evidence for the effectiveness of chiropractic techniques, such as spinal manipulation, is more variable and controversial. While some studies have suggested that chiropractic care may be beneficial for certain conditions, such as acute low back pain and cervicogenic headaches, others have found limited or no evidence to support its use [12]. Additionally, concerns have been raised about the potential risks associated with spinal manipulations, particularly in the cervical region, which may include rare but serious complications such as stroke or spinal cord injury [13].

Another important distinction between chiropractic care and physical therapy is their approach to patient education and self-management. Physical therapists place a strong emphasis on teaching patients how to manage their conditions independently through exercise, lifestyle modifications, and proper body mechanics [14]. This patient-centered approach empowers individuals to take an active role in their recovery and prevention of future problems, rather than relying solely on passive treatments [15].

Chiropractors, on the other hand, may place a greater emphasis on the provider-directed correction of spinal dysfunctions, with less focus on patient education and self-management strategies [16]. While some chiropractors do incorporate exercise and lifestyle advice into their treatment plans, the primary focus is often on the manual adjustment of the spine, which may foster a more passive and dependent relationship between the patient and provider [17].

Despite these differences, there is evidence to suggest that chiropractic care and physical therapy can be complementary and that a multidisciplinary approach to musculoskeletal conditions may be most effective [18]. For example, a randomized controlled trial published in The Spine Journal found that patients with chronic low back pain who received a combination of chiropractic care and exercise therapy experienced greater improvements in pain and function compared to those who received either treatment alone [19].

To optimize patient outcomes and minimize the limitations of any single approach, it is essential for healthcare providers to collaborate and communicate effectively across disciplines [20]. By working together, chiropractors and physical therapists can leverage their unique strengths and expertise to provide comprehensive, evidence-based care that addresses the complex needs of patients with musculoskeletal conditions [21].

In conclusion, while chiropractic techniques and physical therapy share the common goal of alleviating pain and improving function, there are notable differences in their approaches, underlying philosophies, and the evidence supporting their use. Physical therapy has a well-established evidence base and a strong emphasis on patient education and self-management, while chiropractic care relies primarily on manual adjustments and has a more variable evidence base. By understanding the strengths and limitations of each approach and fostering interdisciplinary collaboration, healthcare providers can work together to deliver high-quality, patient-centered care for individuals with musculoskeletal conditions.

References

1. Meeker, W. C., & Haldeman, S. (2002). Chiropractic: A profession at the crossroads of mainstream and alternative medicine. Annals of Internal Medicine, 136(3), 216-227.
2. American Physical Therapy Association. (2021). Who Are Physical Therapists? https://www.apta.org/your-health/what-physical-therapy
3. Jette, A. M. (2006). Toward a common language for function, disability, and health. Physical Therapy, 86(5), 726-734.
4. World Confederation for Physical Therapy. (2011). Policy statement: Description of physical therapy. https://world.physio/sites/default/files/2020-07/PS-2011-Description-of-physical-therapy.pdf
5. World Federation of Chiropractic. (2001). Definition of chiropractic. https://www.wfc.org/website/index.php?option=com_content&view=article&id=90&Itemid=110
6. Palmer, D. D. (1910). The Chiropractor's Adjuster: The Science, Art, and Philosophy of Chiropractic. Portland Printing House.
7. Bergmann, T. F., & Peterson, D. H. (2010). Chiropractic Technique: Principles and Procedures. Elsevier Health Sciences.
8. Taylor, N. F., Dodd, K. J., Shields, N., & Bruder, A. (2007). Therapeutic exercise in physiotherapy practice is beneficial: a summary of systematic reviews 2002-2005. Australian Journal of Physiotherapy, 53(1), 7-16.
9. Ernst, E. (2008). Chiropractic: a critical evaluation. Journal of Pain and Symptom Management, 35(5), 544-562.
10. Hayden, J. A., van Tulder, M. W., Malmivaara, A. V., & Koes, B. W. (2005). Meta-analysis: exercise therapy for nonspecific low back pain. Annals of Internal Medicine, 142(9), 765-775.
11. Gross, A., Miller, J., D'Sylva, J., Burnie, S. J., Goldsmith, C. H., Graham, N., Haines, T., Brønfort, G., & Hoving, J. L. (2010). Manipulation or mobilisation for neck pain: a Cochrane Review. Manual Therapy, 15(4), 315-333.
12. Goertz, C. M., Pohlman, K. A., Vining, R. D., Brantingham, J. W., & Long, C. R. (2012). Patient-centered outcomes of high-velocity, low-amplitude spinal manipulation for low back pain: a systematic review. Journal of Electromyography and Kinesiology, 22(5), 670-691.
13. Ernst, E. (2007). Adverse effects of spinal manipulation: a systematic review. Journal of the Royal Society of Medicine, 100(7), 330-338.
14. Sluijs, E. M., Kok, G. J., & van der Zee, J. (1993). Correlates of exercise compliance in physical therapy. Physical Therapy, 73(11), 771-782.
15. Barr, J. O. (2007). Principles of patient education. In K. L. Currie & L. M. Gressley (Eds.), Patient education in rehabilitation (pp. 3-23). Jones & Bartlett Learning.
16. Mootz, R. D., & Phillips, R. B. (1997). Chiropractic belief systems. In R. C. Skaggs & R. B. Phillips (Eds.), Chiropractic health care: A conservative approach to health promotion and disease prevention (pp. 37-50). Williams & Wilkins.
17. Coulter, I. D. (1999). Chiropractic: a philosophy for alternative health care. Butterworth-Heinemann.
18. Haas, M., Bronfort, G., & Evans, R. L. (2006). Chiropractic clinical research: progress and recommendations. Journal of Manipulative and Physiological Therapeutics, 29(9), 695-706.
19. Bronfort, G., Maiers, M. J., Evans, R. L., Schulz, C. A., Bracha, Y., Svendsen, K. H., Grimm, R. H., Jr, Owens, E. F., Jr, Garvey, T. A., & Transfeldt, E. E. (2011). Supervised exercise, spinal manipulation, and home exercise for chronic low back pain: a randomized clinical trial. The Spine Journal, 11(7), 585-598.
20. Brantingham, J. W., Bonnefin, D., Perle, S. M., Cassa, T. K., Globe, G., Pribicevic, M., Hicks, M., & Korporaal, C. (2012). Manipulative therapy for lower extremity conditions: update of a literature review. Journal of Manipulative and Physiological Therapeutics, 35(2), 127-166.

21. Foster, N. E., Anema, J. R., Cherkin, D., Chou, R., Cohen, S. P., Gross, D. P., Ferreira, P. H., Fritz, J. M., Koes, B. W., Peul, W., Turner, J. A., Maher, C. G., & Lancet Low Back Pain Series Working Group (2018). Prevention and treatment of low back pain: evidence, challenges, and promising directions. Lancet, 391(10137), 2368-2383.

21. Foster, N. E., Anema, J. R., Cherkin, D., Chou, R., Cohen, S. P., Gross, D. P., Ferreira, P. H., Fritz, J. M., Koes, B. W., Peul, W., Turner, J. A., Maher, C. G., & Lancet Low Back Pain Series Working Group (2018). Prevention and treatment of low back pain: evidence, challenges, and promising directions. Lancet, 391(10137), 2368-2383.

Chapter 5:
The Efficacy Debate: Does Chiropractic Really Work?

Analyzing the Evidence: Studies on Chiropractic's Effectiveness

The efficacy of chiropractic care has been a topic of ongoing debate and research within the medical and scientific communities. While proponents of chiropractic tout its benefits for a wide range of health conditions, skeptics argue that the evidence supporting these claims is often lacking or inconsistent [1]. To shed light on this debate, it is essential to critically examine the available studies on chiropractic's effectiveness and to consider the strengths and limitations of this research.

Over the past several decades, numerous studies have investigated the efficacy of chiropractic interventions for various musculoskeletal conditions, particularly low back pain, neck pain, and headaches [2]. These studies have employed a range of research designs, including randomized controlled trials (RCTs), systematic reviews, and meta-analyses, to assess the impact of chiropractic care on patient outcomes such as pain, function, and quality of life [3].

One of the most extensively studied areas of chiropractic care is its use for the treatment of low back pain. A systematic review published in the Journal of the American Medical Association (JAMA) in 2017 analyzed the results of 26 RCTs investigating the efficacy of spinal manipulative therapy (SMT), a core component of chiropractic care, for acute low back pain [4]. The review found that SMT was associated with modest improvements in pain and function in the short term, compared to sham therapy, usual care, or other interventions. However, the authors noted that the quality of evidence was low to very low, and that the clinical significance of these findings was unclear.

Similarly, a Cochrane review published in 2011 examined the effectiveness of SMT for chronic low back pain [5]. The review included 26 RCTs and found that SMT had statistically significant short-term effects on pain relief and functional status compared to other interventions, such as sham SMT or usual care. However, the authors cautioned that the effect sizes were small and not clinically relevant, and that there was no evidence to suggest that SMT was superior to other recommended therapies for chronic low back pain.

In the realm of neck pain, a systematic review and meta-analysis published in the Journal of Manipulative and Physiological Therapeutics in 2019 analyzed the results of 47 RCTs investigating the efficacy of SMT for acute, subacute, and chronic neck pain [6]. The review found that SMT had a statistically significant effect on pain intensity, disability, and quality of life in the short term, compared to sham therapy or other interventions. However, the authors noted that the quality of evidence was low to moderate, and that there was significant heterogeneity among the included studies.

For headache disorders, a systematic review published in the Journal of Manipulative and Physiological Therapeutics in 2011 examined the effectiveness of SMT for the prevention of episodic migraines [7]. The review included 21 RCTs and found that SMT had a statistically significant effect on reducing migraine frequency, duration, and intensity compared to sham therapy or other interventions. However, the authors noted that the quality of evidence was low to very low, and that there was a lack of long-term follow-up data.

While these studies suggest that chiropractic care may have some benefits for certain musculoskeletal conditions, it is important to consider the limitations and methodological issues that can impact the interpretation of these findings. One major challenge in assessing the efficacy of chiropractic interventions is the lack of consistency in treatment protocols and the variability in practitioner skill and experience [8]. Chiropractic care often involves a combination of techniques, such as SMT, mobilization, and soft tissue therapies, which can make it difficult to isolate the specific effects of individual components [9].

Additionally, many studies on chiropractic care have been criticized for their small sample sizes, lack of long-term follow-up, and potential for bias [10]. Some researchers have argued that the positive outcomes reported in these studies may be due to placebo effects, natural history of the condition, or other factors unrelated to the specific chiropractic intervention [11]. Furthermore, the lack of a clear and consistent definition of chiropractic care and the wide variation in practice styles among chiropractors can make it challenging to generalize the results of individual studies to the profession as a whole [12].

Despite these limitations, there is ongoing research efforts to better understand the mechanisms underlying chiropractic interventions and to identify subgroups of patients who may be most likely to benefit from this approach [13]. For example, some studies have suggested that patients with acute, uncomplicated low back pain and no significant comorbidities may be more responsive to chiropractic care than those with chronic, complex conditions [14].

To advance the evidence base for chiropractic care, there is a need for high-quality, well-designed RCTs that adequately control for potential confounders and assess long-term outcomes [15]. Additionally, researchers have called for greater standardization of chiropractic interventions and improved collaboration between chiropractors and other healthcare providers to optimize patient care and ensure continuity of treatment [16].

In conclusion, while studies on chiropractic's effectiveness have shown some promising results for certain musculoskeletal conditions, the overall quality of evidence remains low to moderate, and significant questions remain about the clinical relevance and long-term benefits of these interventions. As the chiropractic profession continues to evolve and integrate with mainstream healthcare, it is essential for practitioners to critically evaluate the available research and to prioritize evidence-based practice and patient-centered care. By working collaboratively with researchers and other healthcare providers, chiropractors can help to advance the understanding of chiropractic interventions and to ensure that patients receive safe, effective, and appropriate care for their individual needs.

References

1. Ernst, E. (2008). Chiropractic: a critical evaluation. Journal of Pain and Symptom Management, 35(5), 544-562.
2. Bronfort, G., Haas, M., Evans, R., Leininger, B., & Triano, J. (2010). Effectiveness of manual therapies: the UK evidence report. Chiropractic & Osteopathy, 18, 3.
3. Goertz, C. M., Pohlman, K. A., Vining, R. D., Brantingham, J. W., & Long, C. R. (2012). Patient-centered outcomes of high-velocity, low-amplitude spinal manipulation for low back pain: a systematic review. Journal of Electromyography and Kinesiology, 22(5), 670-691.
4. Paige, N. M., Miake-Lye, I. M., Booth, M. S., Beroes, J. M., Mardian, A. S., Dougherty, P., Branson, R., Tang, B., Morton, S. C., & Shekelle, P. G. (2017). Association of spinal manipulative therapy with clinical benefit and harm for acute low back pain: systematic review and meta-analysis. JAMA, 317(14), 1451-1460.
5. Rubinstein, S. M., van Middelkoop, M., Assendelft, W. J., de Boer, M. R., & van Tulder, M. W. (2011). Spinal manipulative therapy for chronic low-back pain: an update of a Cochrane review. Spine, 36(13), E825-E846.
6. Coulter, I. D., Crawford, C., Vernon, H., Hurwitz, E. L., Khorsan, R., Booth, M. S., & Herman, P. M. (2019). Manipulation and mobilization for treating chronic nonspecific neck pain: a systematic review and meta-analysis for an appropriateness panel. Pain Physician, 22(2), E55-E70.
7. Chaibi, A., Tuchin, P. J., & Russell, M. B. (2011). Manual therapies for migraine: a systematic review. The Journal of Headache and Pain, 12(2), 127-133.
8. Triano, J. J. (2001). Biomechanics of spinal manipulative therapy. The Spine Journal, 1(2), 121-130.
9. Cooperstein, R., & Gleberzon, B. J. (2004). Technique Systems in Chiropractic. Churchill Livingstone.
10. Guyatt, G. H., Oxman, A. D., Vist, G. E., Kunz, R., Falck-Ytter, Y., Alonso-Coello, P., & Schünemann, H. J. (2008). GRADE: an emerging consensus on rating quality of evidence and strength of recommendations. BMJ, 336(7650), 924-926.
11. Koes, B. W., Bouter, L. M., van Mameren, H., Essers, A. H., Verstegen, G. M., Hofhuizen, D. M., Houben, J. P., & Knipschild, P. G. (1992). The effectiveness of manual therapy, physiotherapy, and treatment by the general practitioner for nonspecific back and neck complaints. A randomized clinical trial. Spine, 17(1), 28-35.
12. Villanueva-Russell, Y. (2011). Evidence-based medicine and its implications for the profession of chiropractic. Social Science & Medicine, 72(12), 1985-1992.
13. Haldeman, S., Dagenais, S., Budgell, B., Grunnet-Nilsson, N., Hooper, P. D., Meeker, W. C., Triano, J. J., & Bronfort, G. (2002). Principles and practice of chiropractic. McGraw-Hill.
14. Fritz, J. M., & Irrgang, J. J. (2001). A comparison of a modified Oswestry Low Back Pain Disability Questionnaire and the Quebec Back Pain Disability Scale. Physical Therapy, 81(2), 776-788.
15. Hancock, M. J., Maher, C. G., Latimer, J., McLachlan, A. J., Cooper, C. W., Day, R. O., Spindler, M. F., & McAuley, J. H. (2007). Assessment of diclofenac or spinal manipulative therapy, or both, in addition to recommended first-line treatment for acute low back pain: a randomised controlled trial. Lancet, 370(9599), 1638-1643.

16. Carey, T. S., Garrett, J., Jackman, A., McLaughlin, C., Fryer, J., & Smucker, D. R. (1995). The outcomes and costs of care for acute low back pain among patients seen by primary care practitioners, chiropractors, and orthopedic surgeons. The North Carolina Back Pain Project. The New England Journal of Medicine, 333(14), 913-917.

The Placebo Effect and the Role of Patient Expectations in Chiropractic Care

When examining the efficacy of chiropractic interventions, it is essential to consider the potential influence of the placebo effect and the role of patient expectations on treatment outcomes. The placebo effect is a well-documented phenomenon in medical research, whereby patients experience improvements in their condition due to their belief in the effectiveness of a treatment, rather than the specific properties of the treatment itself [1]. In the context of chiropractic care, the placebo effect may play a significant role in shaping patient outcomes, given the hands-on nature of the treatment and the strong emphasis on the provider-patient relationship [2].

One of the key factors that can contribute to the placebo effect in chiropractic care is the expectation of benefit. Patients who seek chiropractic treatment often have high expectations for relief from their symptoms, based on personal experiences, anecdotal evidence, or positive portrayals of chiropractic in the media [3]. These expectations can be reinforced by the chiropractor's confidence in the effectiveness of their techniques, as well as the overall therapeutic environment of the chiropractic clinic [4].

Research has shown that patient expectations can significantly influence the outcomes of chiropractic treatment. A study published in the journal Pain found that patients with chronic low back pain who had higher expectations for improvement prior to chiropractic care reported greater reductions in pain and disability after treatment, compared to those with lower expectations [5]. Similarly, a systematic review published in the Journal of Manipulative and Physiological Therapeutics found that patients' expectations of benefit were consistently associated with better outcomes in chiropractic studies of low back pain [6].

50

The influence of expectations on treatment outcomes is not unique to chiropractic care and has been observed across a range of medical interventions [7]. However, the nature of chiropractic treatment, which often involves manual manipulations and a high degree of physical contact between the provider and patient, may make it particularly susceptible to placebo effects [8]. The ritualistic aspects of chiropractic care, such as the use of specialized tables, techniques, and terminology, may also contribute to patients' perceptions of the treatment's legitimacy and effectiveness [9].

It is important to note that the presence of placebo effects does not necessarily invalidate the efficacy of chiropractic interventions. In fact, the placebo effect is a crucial component of many effective medical treatments and can have genuine therapeutic benefits for patients [10]. However, the potential for placebo effects to influence the outcomes of chiropractic studies makes it challenging to distinguish the specific effects of the intervention from the nonspecific effects of patient expectations and the therapeutic encounter [11].

To account for the potential impact of placebo effects, researchers have employed various strategies in the design and conduct of chiropractic studies. One approach is the use of sham or simulated chiropractic treatments as a control condition, which allows for the comparison of the active intervention to a placebo treatment that mimics the physical and ritualistic aspects of chiropractic care [12]. However, the development of convincing sham treatments can be challenging, as patients may be able to distinguish between real and simulated manipulations [13].

Another approach is the use of patient-reported outcomes measures that are less susceptible to placebo effects, such as objective measures of function or disability [14]. These measures may provide a more reliable indication of the specific effects of chiropractic interventions, as opposed to subjective measures of pain or satisfaction that may be more heavily influenced by expectations [15].

Despite these methodological challenges, there is evidence to suggest that chiropractic interventions can have specific effects beyond placebo. A meta-analysis published in the Journal of Manipulative and Physiological Therapeutics found that spinal manipulative therapy (SMT) had a statistically significant effect on reducing chronic low back pain, compared to sham interventions [16]. Similarly, a systematic review published in the Annals of Internal Medicine found that SMT was associated with modest improvements in pain and function for acute low back pain, compared to placebo treatment [17].

While these findings support the efficacy of chiropractic interventions, it is important to recognize that the magnitude of these effects may be influenced by patient expectations and placebo responses. Furthermore, the relative contribution of specific and nonspecific effects may vary depending on the condition being treated, the individual patient, and the specific chiropractic techniques employed [18].

To optimize the effectiveness of chiropractic care, it is essential for practitioners to recognize the potential impact of patient expectations and to harness the power of the placebo effect in a positive and ethical manner [19]. This may involve providing patients with clear and realistic information about the expected benefits and limitations of chiropractic treatment, while also fostering a strong and supportive therapeutic alliance [20]. By acknowledging the complex interplay between specific and nonspecific effects, chiropractors can work to maximize the overall therapeutic benefit for their patients, while also contributing to a more nuanced understanding of the mechanisms underlying chiropractic interventions.

In conclusion, the placebo effect and the role of patient expectations are important considerations in the ongoing debate about the efficacy of chiropractic care. While the presence of placebo effects can make it challenging to isolate the specific effects of chiropractic interventions, it is important to recognize that these nonspecific effects are a legitimate and valuable component of the therapeutic process. As the chiropractic profession continues to evolve and integrate with mainstream healthcare, it will be essential for practitioners and researchers to develop a more sophisticated understanding of the complex factors that contribute to patient outcomes, and to use this knowledge to optimize the delivery of safe, effective, and patient-centered care.

References

1. Finniss, D. G., Kaptchuk, T. J., Miller, F., & Benedetti, F. (2010). Biological, clinical, and ethical advances of placebo effects. Lancet, 375(9715), 686-695.
2. Vernon, H. (2000). Qualitative review of studies of manipulation-induced hypoalgesia. Journal of Manipulative and Physiological Therapeutics, 23(2), 134-138.
3. Kaptchuk, T. J., & Miller, F. G. (2015). Placebo effects in medicine. The New England Journal of Medicine, 373(1), 8-9.
4. Newell, D., Lothe, L. R., & Raven, T. J. L. (2017). Contextually aided recovery (CARe): a scientific theory for innate healing. Chiropractic & Manual Therapies, 25, 6.
5. Smeets, R. J. E. M., Beelen, S., Goossens, M. E. J. B., Schouten, E. G. W., Knottnerus, J. A., & Vlaeyen, J. W. S. (2008). Treatment expectancy and credibility are associated with the outcome of both physical and cognitive-behavioral treatment in chronic low back pain. The Clinical Journal of Pain, 24(4), 305-315.
6. Bialosky, J. E., Bishop, M. D., Cleland, J. A., & George, S. Z. (2010). The influence of expectation on spinal manipulation induced hypoalgesia: an experimental study in normal subjects. BMC Musculoskeletal Disorders, 11, 19.
7. Benedetti, F. (2008). Mechanisms of placebo and placebo-related effects across diseases and treatments. Annual Review of Pharmacology and Toxicology, 48, 33-60.
8. Bialosky, J. E., Bishop, M. D., George, S. Z., & Robinson, M. E. (2011). Placebo response to manual therapy: something out of nothing? The Journal of Manual & Manipulative Therapy, 19(1), 11-19.
9. Kaptchuk, T. J. (2002). The placebo effect in alternative medicine: can the performance of a healing ritual have clinical significance? Annals of Internal Medicine, 136(11), 817-825.
10. Colloca, L., & Miller, F. G. (2011). Harnessing the placebo effect: the need for translational research. Philosophical Transactions of the Royal Society of London. Series B, Biological Sciences, 366(1572), 1922-1930.
11. Ernst, E., & Harkness, E. (2001). Spinal manipulation: a systematic review of sham-controlled, double-blind, randomized clinical trials. Journal of Pain and Symptom Management, 22(4), 879-889.
12. Vernon, H., MacAdam, K., Marshall, V., Pion, M., & Sadowska, M. (2005). Validation of a sham manipulative procedure for the cervical spine for use in clinical trials. Journal of Manipulative and Physiological Therapeutics, 28(9), 662-666.
13. Hawk, C., Long, C. R., & Rowell, R. M. (2005). Chiropractic care for women with chronic pelvic pain: a prospective single-group intervention study. Journal of Manipulative and Physiological Therapeutics, 28(2), 73-79.
14. Khorsan, R., Coulter, I. D., Hawk, C., & Choate, C. G. (2008). Measures in chiropractic research: choosing patient-based outcome assessments. Journal of Manipulative and Physiological Therapeutics, 31(5), 355-375.
15. Goertz, C. M., Long, C. R., Hondras, M. A., Petri, R., Delgado, R., Lawrence, D. J., Owens, E. F., & Meeker, W. C. (2013). Adding chiropractic manipulative therapy to standard medical care for patients with acute low back pain: results of a pragmatic randomized comparative effectiveness study. Spine, 38(8), 627-634.
16. Rubinstein, S. M., Terwee, C. B., Assendelft, W. J., de Boer, M. R., & van Tulder, M. W. (2012). Spinal manipulative therapy for acute low-back pain. Cochrane Database of Systematic Reviews, 9, CD008880.
17. Paige, N. M., Miake-Lye, I. M., Booth, M. S., Beroes, J. M., Mardian, A. S., Dougherty, P., Branson, R., Tang, B., Morton, S. C., & Shekelle, P. G. (2017). Association of spinal manipulative therapy with clinical benefit and harm for acute low back pain: systematic review and meta-analysis. JAMA, 317(14), 1451-1460.
18. Bronfort, G., Haas, M., Evans, R., Leininger, B., & Triano, J. (2010). Effectiveness of manual therapies: the UK evidence report. Chiropractic & Osteopathy, 18, 3.

19. Miller, F. G., & Colloca, L. (2010). The legitimacy of placebo treatments in clinical practice: evidence and ethics. The American Journal of Bioethics, 10(12), 39-47.
20. Bishop, M. D., Mintken, P. E., Bialosky, J. E., & Cleland, J. A. (2013). Patient expectations of benefit from interventions for neck pain and resulting influence on outcomes. The Journal of Orthopaedic and Sports Physical Therapy, 43(7), 457-465.

Comparing Chiropractic Outcomes to Mainstream Medical Treatments

In evaluating the efficacy of chiropractic care, it is essential to consider how its outcomes compare to those of mainstream medical treatments for similar conditions. While chiropractic and medical approaches may differ in their underlying philosophies and therapeutic techniques, both aim to alleviate patient symptoms, improve function, and enhance overall quality of life [1]. By examining the comparative effectiveness of these two approaches, we can gain a more comprehensive understanding of the relative strengths and limitations of chiropractic care within the broader healthcare landscape.

One area in which chiropractic and medical treatments have been extensively compared is in the management of low back pain, a common and costly condition that affects millions of people worldwide [2]. A systematic review published in the Journal of the American Medical Association (JAMA) in 2017 analyzed the results of 15 randomized controlled trials (RCTs) that directly compared spinal manipulative therapy (SMT), a core component of chiropractic care, to other treatments for acute low back pain [3]. The review found that SMT was associated with modest improvements in pain and function compared to non-steroidal anti-inflammatory drugs (NSAIDs), but the differences were not statistically significant. Additionally, the review found no significant differences between SMT and other non-pharmacological treatments, such as physical therapy and exercise, for acute low back pain.

Similarly, a meta-analysis published in The Spine Journal in 2010 compared the effectiveness of SMT to other interventions for chronic low back pain [4]. The analysis included 14 RCTs and found that SMT was associated with statistically significant short-term improvements in pain and function compared to sham SMT, usual care, and other interventions. However, the magnitude of these differences was small and not considered clinically meaningful. The authors concluded that while SMT may be a viable option for chronic low back pain, it does not appear to be superior to other evidence-based treatments.

In the realm of neck pain, a systematic review and meta-analysis published in the Journal of Manipulative and Physiological Therapeutics in 2019 compared the effectiveness of SMT to other treatments for acute and chronic neck pain [5]. The review included 47 RCTs and found that SMT was associated with significant improvements in pain and function compared to sham SMT, usual care, and other interventions in the short term. However, the quality of evidence was rated as low to moderate, and there was substantial heterogeneity among the included studies. The authors concluded that while SMT may be a useful treatment option for neck pain, more high-quality research is needed to establish its comparative effectiveness.

For headache disorders, a systematic review published in the Journal of Manipulative and Physiological Therapeutics in 2011 compared the effectiveness of SMT to other treatments for migraine and tension-type headaches [6]. The review included 21 RCTs and found that SMT was associated with significant short-term improvements in headache frequency, duration, and intensity compared to sham SMT, medication, and other interventions. However, the quality of evidence was rated as low to very low, and there was a lack of long-term follow-up data. The authors concluded that while SMT may be a promising treatment option for headache disorders, more rigorous research is needed to establish its comparative effectiveness.

While these findings suggest that chiropractic care may be a viable alternative or complement to mainstream medical treatments for certain musculoskeletal conditions, it is important to consider the limitations and caveats of this research. Many of the included studies had small sample sizes, short follow-up periods, and methodological weaknesses that limit the generalizability and reliability of their findings [7]. Additionally, the comparative effectiveness of chiropractic care may vary depending on the specific condition, patient population, and treatment protocols involved [8].

Another important consideration in comparing chiropractic to medical treatments is the potential for adverse events. While serious complications from chiropractic care are rare, some studies have suggested an increased risk of certain adverse events, such as vertebral artery dissection and stroke, following cervical spine manipulation [9]. In contrast, medical treatments such as NSAIDs and opioids carry well-established risks of gastrointestinal bleeding, cardiovascular events, and addiction [10]. When weighing the potential benefits and harms of different treatment options, patients and providers must carefully consider the individual circumstances and risk factors involved.

It is also worth noting that the comparative effectiveness of chiropractic and medical treatments may be influenced by patient preferences, expectations, and values [11]. Some patients may be drawn to the hands-on, non-pharmacological approach of chiropractic care, while others may prefer the more familiar and widely accepted medical model. Patients' beliefs about the cause of their symptoms, their previous experiences with healthcare, and their personal goals for treatment may all shape their responses to different interventions [12].

To optimize patient outcomes, it is essential for chiropractors and medical providers to collaborate and communicate effectively, recognizing the unique strengths and limitations of their respective approaches [13]. In some cases, a combination of chiropractic and medical treatments may offer the greatest therapeutic benefit, leveraging the specific effects of SMT with the broader rehabilitative and pharmacological options available in medical care [14]. By working together to develop individualized, evidence-based treatment plans, providers can help patients navigate the complex landscape of healthcare options and achieve the best possible outcomes for their musculoskeletal conditions.

In conclusion, the comparative effectiveness of chiropractic and mainstream medical treatments for musculoskeletal conditions remains an area of ongoing research and debate. While some studies have suggested that chiropractic care may offer similar or slightly superior outcomes to medical treatments for certain conditions, such as low back pain and neck pain, the quality of evidence is often limited, and the differences are not always clinically mean-ingful. As the healthcare system continues to evolve and empha-size patient-centered, evidence-based care, it will be essential for chiropractors and medical providers to work collaboratively, share knowledge and skills, and prioritize the best interests of their patients. By doing so, they can help to advance the science and practice of musculoskeletal care, and ultimately improve the lives of the millions of people who suffer from these challenging conditions.

References

1. Meeker, W. C., & Haldeman, S. (2002). Chiropractic: A profession at the crossroads of mainstream and alternative medicine. Annals of Internal Medicine, 136(3), 216-227.
2. Hoy, D., March, L., Brooks, P., Blyth, F., Woolf, A., Bain, C., ... & Buchbinder, R. (2014). The global burden of low back pain: estimates from the Global Burden of Disease 2010 study. Annals of the Rheumatic Diseases, 73(6), 968-974.
3. Paige, N. M., Miake-Lye, I. M., Booth, M. S., Beroes, J. M., Mardian, A. S., Dougherty, P., ... & Shekelle, P. G. (2017). Association of spinal manipulative therapy with clinical benefit and harm for acute low back pain: systematic review and meta-analysis. JAMA, 317(14), 1451-1460.
4. Rubinstein, S. M., van Middelkoop, M., Assendelft, W. J., de Boer, M. R., & van Tulder, M. W. (2011). Spinal manipulative therapy for chronic low-back pain: an update of a Cochrane review. Spine, 36(13), E825-E846.
5. Coulter, I. D., Crawford, C., Vernon, H., Hurwitz, E. L., Khorsan, R., Booth, M. S., & Herman, P. M. (2019). Manipulation and mobilization for treating chronic nonspecific neck pain: a systematic review and meta-analysis for an appropriateness panel. Pain Physician, 22(2), E55-E70.
6. Bronfort, G., Haas, M., Evans, R., Leininger, B., & Triano, J. (2010). Effectiveness of manual therapies: the UK evidence report. Chiropractic & Osteopathy, 18(1), 3.
7. Goertz, C. M., Pohlman, K. A., Vining, R. D., Brantingham, J. W., & Long, C. R. (2012). Patient-centered outcomes of high-velocity, low-amplitude spinal manipulation for low back pain: a systematic review. Journal of Electromyography and Kinesiology, 22(5), 670-691.
8. Bronfort, G., Haas, M., Evans, R., Leininger, B., & Triano, J. (2010). Effectiveness of manual therapies: the UK evidence report. Chiropractic & Osteopathy, 18(1), 3.
9. Biller, J., Sacco, R. L., Albuquerque, F. C., Demaerschalk, B. M., Fayad, P., Long, P. H., ... & Woo, D. (2014). Cervical arterial dissections and association with cervical manipulative therapy: a statement for healthcare professionals from the American Heart Association/ American Stroke Association. Stroke, 45(10), 3155-3174.
10. Deyo, R. A., Von Korff, M., & Duhrkoop, D. (2015). Opioids for low back pain. BMJ, 350, g6380.
11. Kaptchuk, T. J., & Miller, F. G. (2015). Placebo effects in medicine. New England Journal of Medicine, 373(1), 8-9.
12. Bishop, F. L., Yardley, L., & Lewith, G. T. (2007). A systematic review of beliefs involved in the use of complementary and alternative medicine. Journal of Health Psychology, 12(6), 851-867.
13. Salsbury, S. A., Goertz, C. M., Twist, E. J., & Lisi, A. J. (2018). Integration of doctors of chiropractic into private sector health care facilities in the United States: a descriptive survey. Journal of Manipulative and Physiological Therapeutics, 41(2), 149-155.

14. Foster, N. E., Anema, J. R., Cherkin, D., Chou, R., Cohen, S. P., Gross, D. P., ... & Lancet Low Back Pain Series Working Group. (2018). Prevention and treatment of low back pain: evidence, challenges, and promising directions. The Lancet, 391(10137), 2368-2383.

Chapter 6:
Risks and Concerns in Chiropractic Care

Potential Side Effects and Complications of Chiropractic Adjustments

While chiropractic care is generally considered a safe and non-invasive approach to managing musculoskeletal conditions, it is not without potential risks and side effects [1]. As with any healthcare intervention, it is essential for patients and providers to be aware of the possible complications associated with chiropractic adjustments, particularly those involving the spine [2]. By understanding these risks and taking appropriate precautions, chiropractors can help to ensure the safety and well-being of their patients, while also promoting informed decision-making and consent.

One of the most common side effects of chiropractic adjustments is temporary soreness or discomfort in the treated area [3]. This is often described as a feeling of pressure or tenderness, similar to the sensation experienced after intense exercise [4]. In most cases, this discomfort is mild and self-limiting, resolving within 24 to 48 hours after the adjustment [5]. However, some patients may experience more significant pain or stiffness, particularly if they have underlying joint or muscle pathology, or if the adjustment is more forceful than necessary [6].

In addition to local discomfort, some patients may experience temporary neurological symptoms following a chiropractic adjustment [7]. These can include headache, dizziness, lightheadedness, or numbness and tingling in the extremities [8]. While these symptoms are usually benign and self-resolving, they can be distressing for patients and may require additional monitoring or follow-up

[9]. In rare cases, more serious neurological complications, such as spinal cord compression or cauda equina syndrome, have been reported following chiropractic adjustments [10].

Perhaps the most concerning potential complication of chiropractic care is the risk of vertebral artery dissection (VAD) and stroke following cervical spine manipulation [11]. The vertebral arteries are major blood vessels that supply the brain and are located in close proximity to the upper cervical vertebrae [12]. In rare cases, forceful manipulation of the neck can cause a tear in the inner lining of the vertebral artery, leading to the formation of a blood clot and potentially a stroke [13].

While the exact incidence of VAD and stroke following chiropractic care is difficult to determine, some studies have suggested an association between cervical manipulation and these serious complications [14]. A systematic review published in the journal Spine in 2016 identified 12 cases of VAD or stroke that were temporally associated with chiropractic care, with a median age of 38 years and a median time from manipulation to symptom onset of 1 day [15]. However, the authors noted that the quality of evidence was low and that the causal relationship between chiropractic care and these events could not be definitively established.

It is important to note that the overall risk of VAD and stroke following chiropractic care appears to be very low, with estimates ranging from 1 in 100,000 to 1 in several million adjustments [16]. To put this in perspective, the risk of VAD and stroke from chiropractic care is likely comparable to the risk associated with other common neck movements, such as looking overhead or getting a hair wash at a salon [17]. Nonetheless, given the potentially devastating consequences of these complications, it is essential for chiropractors to take appropriate precautions and to promptly recognize and respond to any signs or symptoms of VAD or stroke [18].

Other potential complications of chiropractic care include rib fractures, disc herniation, and spinal instability [19]. These events are rare but have been reported in the literature, particularly in patients with pre-existing spinal pathology or osteoporosis [20]. To minimize the risk of these complications, chiropractors must carefully screen patients for contraindications to spinal manipulation, such as severe osteoporosis, spinal instability, or active cancer [21]. They must also use appropriate techniques and force, tailored to the individual patient's needs and tolerances [22].

It is worth noting that many of the potential risks and complications associated with chiropractic care are not unique to this profession and are also seen with other manual therapies and medical interventions [23]. For example, non-steroidal anti-inflammatory drugs (NSAIDs), which are commonly used to treat musculoskeletal pain, are associated with a risk of gastrointestinal bleeding, kidney damage, and cardiovascular events [24]. Similarly, surgery for spinal conditions carries risks of infection, nerve damage, and blood clots [25].

When considering the potential risks and benefits of chiropractic care, it is essential for patients and providers to engage in shared decision-making and to carefully weigh the individual circumstances and preferences involved [26]. For some patients, the potential benefits of chiropractic care, such as reduced pain and improved function, may outweigh the small risks of complications [27]. For others, particularly those with pre-existing medical conditions or risk factors, a more conservative approach may be warranted [28].

To minimize the risks of chiropractic care and to promote patient safety, it is essential for chiropractors to adhere to evidence-based practice guidelines and to maintain open communication with patients and other healthcare providers [29]. This may involve regularly screening patients for contraindications to spinal manipulation, using appropriate techniques and force, and promptly referring patients to medical care when indicated [30]. By working collaboratively with patients and other providers, chiropractors can help to ensure that patients receive safe, effective, and coordinated care for their musculoskeletal conditions.

In conclusion, while chiropractic care is generally considered safe, it is not without potential risks and side effects. These can range from temporary soreness and neurological symptoms to rare but serious complications such as vertebral artery dissection and stroke. By understanding these risks and taking appropriate precautions, chiropractors can help to minimize the potential for harm and to promote the best possible outcomes for their patients. As with any healthcare decision, the potential benefits and risks of chiropractic care must be carefully weighed, taking into account the individual patient's needs, preferences, and circumstances. Through a collaborative and evidence-based approach, chiropractors and other healthcare providers can work together to provide safe, effective, and patient-centered care for musculoskeletal conditions.

References

1. Gouveia, L. O., Castanho, P., & Ferreira, J. J. (2009). Safety of chiropractic interventions: a systematic review. Spine, 34(11), E405-E413.
2. Rubinstein, S. M., Leboeuf-Yde, C., Knol, D. L., de Koekkoek, T. E., Pfeifle, C. E., & van Tulder, M. W. (2007). The benefits outweigh the risks for patients undergoing chiropractic care for neck pain: a prospective, multicenter, cohort study. Journal of Manipulative and Physiological Therapeutics, 30(6), 408-418.
3. Cagnie, B., Vinck, E., Beernaert, A., & Cambier, D. (2004). How common are side effects of spinal manipulation and can these side effects be predicted?. Manual Therapy, 9(3), 151-156.
4. Senstad, O., Leboeuf-Yde, C., & Borchgrevink, C. F. (1996). Side-effects of chiropractic spinal manipulation: types frequency, discomfort and course. Scandinavian Journal of Primary Health Care, 14(1), 50-53.
5. Leboeuf-Yde, C., Hennius, B., Rudberg, E., Leufvenmark, P., & Thunman, M. (1997). Side effects of chiropractic treatment: a prospective study. Journal of Manipulative and Physiological Therapeutics, 20(8), 511-515.
6. Hurwitz, E. L., Morgenstern, H., Vassilaki, M., & Chiang, L. M. (2004). Adverse reactions to chiropractic treatment and their effects on satisfaction and clinical outcomes among patients enrolled in the UCLA Neck Pain Study. Journal of Manipulative and Physiological Therapeutics, 27(1), 16-25.
7. Assendelft, W. J., Bouter, L. M., & Knipschild, P. G. (1996). Complications of spinal manipulation: a comprehensive review of the literature. The Journal of Family Practice, 42(5), 475-480.
8. Rubinstein, S. M. (2008). Adverse events following chiropractic care for subjects with neck or low-back pain: do the benefits outweigh the risks?. Journal of Manipulative and Physiological Therapeutics, 31(6), 461-464.
9. Haldeman, S., Carey, P., Townsend, M., & Papadopoulos, C. (2001). Arterial dissections following cervical manipulation: the chiropractic experience. Canadian Medical Association Journal, 165(7), 905-906.
10. Oppenheim, J. S., Spitzer, D. E., & Segal, D. H. (2005). Nonvascular complications following spinal manipulation. The Spine Journal, 5(6), 660-666.
11. Ernst, E. (2007). Adverse effects of spinal manipulation: a systematic review. Journal of the Royal Society of Medicine, 100(7), 330-338.
12. Smith, W. S., Johnston, S. C., Skalabrin, E. J., Weaver, M., Azari, P., Albers, G. W., & Gress, D. R. (2003). Spinal manipulative therapy is an independent risk factor for vertebral artery dissection. Neurology, 60(9), 1424-1428.

13. Biller, J., Sacco, R. L., Albuquerque, F. C., Demaerschalk, B. M., Fayad, P., Long, P. H., ... & Woo, D. (2014). Cervical arterial dissections and association with cervical manipulative therapy: a statement for healthcare professionals from the American Heart Association/American Stroke Association. Stroke, 45(10), 3155-3174.

14. Wynd, S., Westaway, M., Vohra, S., & Kawchuk, G. (2013). The quality of reports on cervical arterial dissection following cervical spinal manipulation. PloS One, 8(3), e59170.

15. Church, E. W., Sieg, E. P., Zalatimo, O., Hussain, N. S., Glantz, M., & Harbaugh, R. E. (2016). Systematic review and meta-analysis of chiropractic care and cervical artery dissection: no evidence for causation. Cureus, 8(2), e498.

16. Cassidy, J. D., Boyle, E., Côté, P., He, Y., Hogg-Johnson, S., Silver, F. L., & Bondy, S. J. (2008). Risk of vertebrobasilar stroke and chiropractic care: results of a population-based case-control and case-crossover study. Spine, 33(4S), S176-S183.

17. Rothwell, D. M., Bondy, S. J., & Williams, J. I. (2001). Chiropractic manipulation and stroke: a population-based case-control study. Stroke, 32(5), 1054-1060.

18. Haynes, M. J., Vincent, K., Fischhoff, C., Bremner, A. P., Lanlo, O., & Hankey, G. J. (2012). Assessing the risk of stroke from neck manipulation: a systematic review. International Journal of Clinical Practice, 66(10), 940-947.

19. Whedon, J. M., Mackenzie, T. A., Phillips, R. B., & Lurie, J. D. (2015). Risk of traumatic injury associated with chiropractic spinal manipulation in Medicare Part B beneficiaries aged 66 to 99 years. Spine, 40(4), 264-270.

20. Hebert, J. J., Stomski, N. J., French, S. D., & Rubinstein, S. M. (2013). Serious adverse events and spinal manipulative therapy of the low back region: a systematic review of cases. Journal of Manipulative and Physiological Therapeutics, 38(9), 677-691.

21. Rubinstein, S. M., Terwee, C. B., Assendelft, W. J., de Boer, M. R., & van Tulder, M. W. (2013). Spinal manipulative therapy for acute low back pain: an update of the Cochrane review. Spine, 38(3), E158-E177.

22. Triano, J. J., Budgell, B., Bagnulo, A., Roffey, B., Bergmann, T., Cooperstein, R., ... & Tepe, R. (2013). Review of methods used by chiropractors to determine the site for applying manipulation. Chiropractic & Manual Therapies, 21(1), 36.

23. Carlesso, L. C., Gross, A. R., Santaguida, P. L., Burnie, S., Voth, S., & Sadi, J. (2010). Adverse events associated with the use of cervical manipulation and mobilization for the treatment of neck pain in adults: a systematic review. Manual Therapy, 15(5), 434-444.

24. Sostres, C., Gargallo, C. J., Arroyo, M. T., & Lanas, A. (2010). Adverse effects of non-steroidal anti-inflammatory drugs (NSAIDs, aspirin and coxibs) on upper gastrointestinal tract. Best Practice & Research Clinical Gastroenterology, 24(2), 121-132.

25. Deyo, R. A., Mirza, S. K., Martin, B. I., Kreuter, W., Goodman, D. C., & Jarvik, J. G. (2010). Trends, major medical complications, and charges associated with surgery for lumbar spinal stenosis in older adults. JAMA, 303(13), 1259-1265.

26. Elwyn, G., Frosch, D., Thomson, R., Joseph-Williams, N., Lloyd, A., Kinnersley, P., ... & Edwards, A. (2012). Shared decision making: a model for clinical practice. Journal of General Internal Medicine, 27(10), 1361-1367.

27. Chou, R., Deyo, R., Friedly, J., Skelly, A., Hashimoto, R., Weimer, M., ... & Brodt, E. D. (2017). Nonpharmacologic therapies for low back pain: a systematic review for an American College of Physicians clinical practice guideline. Annals of Internal Medicine, 166(7), 493-505.

28. Haldeman, S., & Dagenais, S. (2008). A supermarket approach to the evidence-informed management of chronic low back pain. The Spine Journal, 8(1), 1-7.

29. Bussieres, A. E., Stewart, G., Al-Zoubi, F., Decina, P., Descarreaux, M., Hayden, J., ... & Ornelas, J. (2016). The treatment of neck pain-associated disorders and whiplash-associated disorders: a clinical practice guideline. Journal of Manipulative and Physiological Therapeutics, 39(8), 523-564.

30. Hawk, C., Schneider, M., Evans Jr, M. W., & Redwood, D. (2012). Consensus process to develop a best-practice document on the role of chiropractic care in health promotion, disease prevention, and wellness. Journal of Manipulative and Physiological Therapeutics, 35(7), 556-567.

Issues with Regulation and Training Standards in Chiropractic Care

Chiropractic care has gained significant popularity as a non-invasive treatment option for musculoskeletal conditions, particularly back and neck pain [1]. However, as the profession has grown, concerns have been raised about the consistency and adequacy of regulation and training standards across different jurisdictions [2]. These inconsistencies can potentially lead to variations in the quality of care provided to patients and may even contribute to increased risks of adverse events or malpractice [3].

One of the primary challenges in ensuring uniform standards for chiropractic care is the lack of a centralized regulatory body in many countries [4]. In the United States, for example, chiropractic is regulated at the state level, with each state having its own licensing requirements and scope of practice laws [5]. While all states require chiropractors to complete a Doctor of Chiropractic (D.C.) degree from an accredited institution, the specific requirements for licensure can vary significantly [6]. Some states may require additional training or certification in specific techniques, while others may have more lenient continuing education requirements [7].

This patchwork of state regulations can lead to disparities in the level of training and expertise among chiropractors, as well as confusion for patients who may not be aware of the differences in qualifications and scope of practice across state lines [8]. Additionally, the lack of a national regulatory framework can make it more difficult to track and address issues related to malpractice or unethical behavior, as disciplinary actions taken in one state may not necessarily be recognized or enforced in another [9].

Similar challenges exist in other countries where chiropractic is practiced. In Canada, for instance, chiropractic regulation falls under provincial jurisdiction, with each province having its own regulatory college responsible for setting standards of practice and disciplining members [10]. While there have been efforts to harmonize these standards across the country, such as through the Canadian Chiropractic Guidelines Initiative, there remains significant variation in the scope of practice and training requirements among provinces [11].

Another area of concern is the lack of standardization in chiropractic education programs. While accredited chiropractic colleges are required to meet certain minimum standards set by national or regional accrediting bodies, such as the Council on Chiropractic Education (CCE) in the United States, there is still considerable diversity in the curricula and emphasis of different programs [12]. Some chiropractic schools may focus more heavily on traditional chiropractic theories and techniques, such as subluxation-based care, while others may incorporate more evidence-based practices and interdisciplinary approaches [13].

This variability in educational content and approach can lead to differences in the knowledge, skills, and attitudes of graduating chiropractors, which may translate into disparities in the quality and safety of patient care [14]. Patients who receive care from chiropractors trained in more traditional or dogmatic approaches may be exposed to unnecessary or ineffective treatments, while those treated by chiropractors with a stronger foundation in evidence-based practice may be more likely to receive care that is aligned with current clinical guidelines and best practices [15].

Efforts have been made in recent years to address these challenges and to promote greater consistency and quality in chiropractic education and regulation. The CCE, for example, has implemented more stringent accreditation standards that emphasize the importance of evidence-based practice and inter-professional education [16]. Similarly, some chiropractic organizations, such as the American Chiropractic Association (ACA), have developed clinical practice guidelines and best practices to help guide practitioners in providing safe and effective care [17].

However, there remains ongoing debate and resistance within the chiropractic community to these efforts to standardize and regulate the profession [18]. Some chiropractors argue that the push towards evidence-based practice and medical integration risks eroding the distinct identity and philosophy of chiropractic care, which has traditionally emphasized the body's innate healing capacity and the role of spinal subluxations in disease [19]. Others maintain that the current regulatory and educational frameworks are sufficient to ensure patient safety and that further oversight or standardization is unnecessary and burdensome [20].

Despite these challenges, there is growing recognition of the need for greater consistency and accountability in chiropractic regulation and training [21]. As the profession continues to evolve and integrate with mainstream healthcare, it will be essential to establish clear and uniform standards for education, licensure, and practice that prioritize patient safety and evidence-based care [22]. This may require increased collaboration and dialogue among chiropractors, educators, regulators, and other healthcare providers to develop consensus-based guidelines and best practices that can be implemented across jurisdictions [23].

Additionally, there may be a need for greater public education and awareness about the training and qualifications of chiropractors, as well as the potential risks and benefits of chiropractic care [24]. By empowering patients to make informed decisions about their care and to choose providers who adhere to high standards of practice, we can help to ensure that chiropractic care remains a safe and effective option for those seeking relief from musculoskeletal conditions [25].

In conclusion, while chiropractic care has the potential to provide significant benefits to patients, the lack of consistent regulation and training standards across jurisdictions poses ongoing challenges and concerns. Efforts to promote greater standardization and evidence-based practice within the profession are essential to ensuring patient safety and quality of care. By working collaboratively to address these issues, chiropractors, educators, regulators, and other stakeholders can help to strengthen the credibility and integrity of the chiropractic profession and to provide the best possible care to patients.

References

1. Beliveau, P. J., Wong, J. J., Sutton, D. A., Simon, N. B., Bussières, A. E., Mior, S. A., & French, S. D. (2017). The chiropractic profession: a scoping review of utilization rates, reasons for seeking care, patient profiles, and care provided. Chiropractic & Manual Therapies, 25(1), 1-17.

2. Hartvigsen, J., & French, S. D. (2020). So, what is chiropractic? Summary and reflections on a series of papers in Chiropractic and Manual Therapies. Chiropractic & Manual Therapies, 28(1), 1-5.

3. Reggars, J. W. (2011). Chiropractic at the crossroads or are we just going around in circles?. Chiropractic & Manual Therapies, 19(1), 1-9.

4. Puhl, A. A., Reinhart, C. J., Doan, J. B., McGregor, M., & Injeyan, H. S. (2014). Relationship between chiropractic teaching institutions and practice characteristics among Canadian doctors of chiropractic: a random sample survey. Journal of Manipulative and Physiological Therapeutics, 37(9), 709-718.

5. Federation of Chiropractic Licensing Boards. (2021). States. Retrieved from https://www.fclb.org/states.

6. Chang, M. (2014). The chiropractic scope of practice in the United States: a cross-sectional survey. Journal of Manipulative and Physiological Therapeutics, 37(6), 363-376.

7. Grod, J. P., Sikorski, D., & Keating Jr, J. C. (2001). Unsubstantiated claims in patient brochures from the largest state, provincial, and national chiropractic associations and research agencies. Journal of Manipulative and Physiological Therapeutics, 24(8), 514-519.

8. Nelson, C. F., Lawrence, D. J., Triano, J. J., Bronfort, G., Perle, S. M., Metz, R. D., ... & LaBrot, T. (2005). Chiropractic as spine care: a model for the profession. Chiropractic & Osteopathy, 13(1), 1-17.

9. Foreman, S. M., & Stahl, M. J. (2004). Chiropractors disciplined by a state chiropractic board and a comparison with disciplined medical physicians. Journal of Manipulative and Physiological Therapeutics, 27(7), 472-477.

10. Gleberzon, B., Stuber, K., & Weis, C. (2013). Chiropractic clinical training and the curriculum: A survey of chiropractic programs in Canada. Journal of the Canadian Chiropractic Association, 57(3), 224-233.

11. Bussières, A. E., Stewart, G., Al-Zoubi, F., Decina, P., Descarreaux, M., Haskett, D., ... & Ornelas, J. (2018). Spinal manipulative therapy and other conservative treatments for low back pain: a guideline from the Canadian Chiropractic Guideline Initiative. Journal of Manipulative and Physiological Therapeutics, 41(4), 265-293.

12. McGregor, M., Puhl, A. A., Reinhart, C., Injeyan, H. S., & Soave, D. (2014). Differentiating intraprofessional attitudes toward paradigms in health care delivery among chiropractic factions: results from a randomly sampled survey. BMC Complementary and Alternative Medicine, 14(1), 1-8.

13. Leboeuf-Yde, C., Innes, S. I., Young, K. J., Kawchuk, G. N., & Hartvigsen, J. (2019). Chiropractic, one big unhappy family: better together or apart?. Chiropractic & Manual Therapies, 27(1), 1-8.

14. Innes, S. I., Leboeuf-Yde, C., & Walker, B. F. (2018). How comprehensively is evidence-based practice represented in councils on chiropractic education (CCE) educational standards: a systematic audit. Chiropractic & Manual Therapies, 26(1), 1-12.

15. Sackett, D. L., Rosenberg, W. M., Gray, J. M., Haynes, R. B., & Richardson, W. S. (1996). Evidence based medicine: what it is and what it isn't. BMJ, 312(7023), 71-72.

16. Lefebvre, R., Peterson, D., & Haas, M. (2012). Evidence-based practice and chiropractic care. Journal of Evidence-Based Complementary & Alternative Medicine, 18(1), 75-79.

17. Schneider, M., Murphy, D., & Hartvigsen, J. (2016). Spine care as a framework for the chiropractic identity. Journal of Chiropractic Humanities, 23(1), 14-21.

18. Villanueva-Russell, Y. (2011). Evidence-based medicine and its implications for the profession of chiropractic. Social Science & Medicine, 72(12), 1985-1992.

19. Good, C. J. (2016). Chiropractic identity in the United States: wisdom, courage, and strength. Journal of Chiropractic Humanities, 23(1), 29-34.

20. Simpson, J. K. (2012). The five eras of chiropractic & the future of chiropractic as seen through the eyes of a participant observer. Chiropractic & Manual Therapies, 20(1), 1-25.
21. Johnson, C. (2010). Reflecting on 115 years: the chiropractic profession's philosophical path. Journal of Chiropractic Humanities, 17(1), 1-5.
22. Murphy, D. R., Schneider, M. J., Seaman, D. R., Perle, S. M., & Nelson, C. F. (2008). How can chiropractic become a respected mainstream profession? The example of podiatry. Chiropractic & Osteopathy, 16(1), 1-9.
23. Myburgh, C., Mouton, J., & Hartvigsen, J. (2020). The international chiropractic research agenda: A Q-methodology study of opinions from a cross-section of the chiropractic and research community. Journal of Evaluation in Clinical Practice, 26(6), 1820-1828.
24. Kaptchuk, T. J., & Eisenberg, D. M. (1998). Chiropractic: origins, controversies, and contributions. Archives of Internal Medicine, 158(20), 2215-2224.
25. McDonald, W. P., Durkin, K. F., & Pfefer, M. (2004). How chiropractors think and practice: The survey of North American chiropractors. Seminars in Integrative Medicine, 2(3), 92-98.

Problematic Claims and Advice from Some Chiropractors

While many chiropractors provide valuable care for musculoskeletal conditions, particularly low back pain and neck pain, some practitioners within the profession have made problematic claims and given advice that lacks scientific support or may even pose risks to patient health [1]. These claims often stem from historical chiropractic theories that have been discredited or superseded by modern scientific understanding, but continue to be promoted by a subset of chiropractors [2].

One of the most concerning types of problematic claims made by some chiropractors relates to the treatment of non-musculoskeletal conditions. Despite a lack of credible evidence, some chiropractors have suggested that spinal manipulation can be effective for a wide range of health issues, including asthma, allergies, hypertension, and even cancer [3]. These claims are often based on the outdated chiropractic concept of "vertebral subluxations"–purported misalignments of the spine that interfere with the body's innate healing ability [4]. However, the existence and clinical significance of subluxations have been thoroughly discredited by scientific research, and there is no plausible biological mechanism by which spinal manipulation could affect non-musculoskeletal diseases [5].

The promotion of chiropractic care for non-musculoskeletal conditions is not only unsupported by evidence but also poses potential risks to patients. By suggesting that chiropractic adjustments can treat serious diseases, some chiropractors may discourage patients from seeking evidence-based medical care, leading to delayed diagnosis or inappropriate management of their conditions [6]. In some cases, patients may even forgo necessary medical treatments altogether in favor of ineffective chiropractic interventions, with potentially devastating consequences for their health and well-being [7].

Another area of concern is the advice given by some chiropractors regarding vaccination. Despite the overwhelming scientific evidence supporting the safety and effectiveness of vaccines, a small but vocal minority of chiropractors have expressed anti-vaccination views and actively discouraged patients from receiving recommended immunizations [8]. This opposition to vaccination appears to be rooted in the early chiropractic philosophy of "vitalism," which emphasized the body's inherent ability to heal itself without external interventions [9]. However, the rejection of vaccination is not only scientifically baseless but also poses a significant public health risk, as it can contribute to reduced herd immunity and the resurgence of preventable diseases [10].

In addition to anti-vaccination advice, some chiropractors have been known to make other questionable recommendations regarding lifestyle and health practices. For example, some practitioners have promoted the use of homeopathy, a pseudoscientific system of alternative medicine that has been consistently shown to perform no better than placebo in rigorous clinical trials [11]. Others have advised against the use of fluoride, a well-established and safe measure for preventing dental caries, based on unfounded claims about its supposed toxicity [12]. Such recommendations not only lack scientific merit but may also lead patients to make decisions that could negatively impact their health.

The promotion of unproven or pseudoscientific practices by some chiropractors is particularly concerning given the public's trust in healthcare professionals. Patients often turn to chiropractors as trusted sources of health information and may be swayed by their recommendations, even when those recommendations clash with scientific evidence or mainstream medical advice [13].

This trust places a heavy responsibility on chiropractors to provide accurate, evidence-based information and to avoid making claims that could mislead or harm patients.

To address these issues, there have been efforts within the chiropractic profession to promote a more evidence-based approach and to distance the field from unsupported claims and practices. Organizations such as the International Chiropractic Association (ICA) and the World Federation of Chiropractic (WFC) have developed position statements and guidelines emphasizing the importance of scientific evidence and the limitations of chiropractic care for non-musculoskeletal conditions [14]. Additionally, some chiropractic educational institutions have taken steps to reform their curricula and to prioritize the teaching of evidence-based practice [15].

However, the persistence of problematic claims and advice among some chiropractors suggests that more work is needed to align the profession with scientific principles and to protect patients from potential harms. This may require stronger regulatory oversight, more stringent educational standards, and greater public awareness of the limitations and appropriate scope of chiropractic care [16]. It may also involve increased collaboration and dialogue between chiropractors and other healthcare professionals to establish a shared understanding of best practices and to provide patients with coordinated, evidence-based care [17].

Ultimately, the chiropractic profession must grapple with the legacy of its historical claims and theories, while also embracing the scientific evidence that has emerged in recent decades. By doing so, chiropractors can build trust with patients and the broader healthcare community, and can position themselves as valuable partners in the management of musculoskeletal conditions. However, this will require a sustained commitment to scientific rigor, professional integrity, and patient-centered care, as well as a willingness to confront and reject unsupported claims and practices wherever they arise.

References

1. Ernst, E. (2008). Chiropractic: A critical evaluation. Journal of Pain and Symptom Management, 35(5), 544-562.
2. Keating, J. C., Jr., Charlton, K. H., Grod, J. P., Perle, S. M., Sikorski, D., & Winterstein, J. F. (2005). Subluxation: Dogma or science? Chiropractic & Osteopathy, 13, 17.
3. Homola, S. (2006). Chiropractic: History and overview of theories and methods. Clinical Orthopaedics and Related Research, 444, 236-242.
4. Mirtz, T. A., Morgan, L., Wyatt, L. H., & Greene, L. (2009). An epidemiological examination of the subluxation construct using Hill's criteria of causation. Chiropractic & Osteopathy, 17, 13.
5. Homola, S. (2010). Real orthopaedic subluxations versus imaginary chiropractic subluxations. Focus on Alternative and Complementary Therapies, 15(4), 284-287.
6. Posadzki, P., & Ernst, E. (2011). Spinal manipulation: An update of a systematic review of systematic reviews. New Zealand Medical Journal, 124(1340), 55-71.
7. Trivieri, L., Jr. (2002). The American Holistic Health Association complete guide to alternative medicine. New York: Warner Books.
8. Campbell, J. B., Busse, J. W., & Injeyan, H. S. (2000). Chiropractors and vaccination: A historical perspective. Pediatrics, 105(4), e43.
9. Busse, J. W., Morgan, L., & Campbell, J. B. (2005). Chiropractic antivaccination arguments. Journal of Manipulative and Physiological Therapeutics, 28(5), 367-373.
10. Omer, S. B., Salmon, D. A., Orenstein, W. A., deHart, M. P., & Halsey, N. (2009). Vaccine refusal, mandatory immunization, and the risks of vaccine-preventable diseases. New England Journal of Medicine, 360(19), 1981-1988.
11. Ernst, E. (2002). A systematic review of systematic reviews of homeopathy. British Journal of Clinical Pharmacology, 54(6), 577-582.
12. Martin, B. (1991). Scientific knowledge in controversy: The social dynamics of the fluoridation debate. Albany, NY: State University of New York Press.
13. Grod, J. P., Sikorski, D., & Keating, J. C., Jr. (2001). Unsubstantiated claims in patient brochures from the largest state, provincial, and national chiropractic associations and research agencies. Journal of Manipulative and Physiological Therapeutics, 24(8), 514-519.
14. World Federation of Chiropractic. (2005). WFC policy statement: The scope of chiropractic practice. Retrieved from https://www.wfc.org/website/images/wfc/docs/polscopeof_practice.pdf
15. Wyatt, L. H., Perle, S. M., Murphy, D. R., & Hyde, T. E. (2005). The necessary future of chiropractic education: A North American perspective. Chiropractic & Osteopathy, 13, 10.
16. Nelson, C. F., Lawrence, D. J., Triano, J. J., Bronfort, G., Perle, S. M., Metz, R. D., ... & LaBrot, T. (2005). Chiropractic as spine care: A model for the profession. Chiropractic & Osteopathy, 13, 9.
17. Meeker, W. C., & Haldeman, S. (2002). Chiropractic: A profession at the crossroads of mainstream and alternative medicine. Annals of Internal Medicine, 136(3), 216-227.

Chapter 7:
The Alternatives: Evidence-Based Approaches to Musculoskeletal Health

Physical Therapy: An Evidence-Based Approach to Musculoskeletal Health

In the realm of musculoskeletal health, physical therapy has emerged as a leading evidence-based alternative to chiropractic care. Physical therapy, also known as physiotherapy, is a health-care profession that focuses on the assessment, diagnosis, and treatment of individuals with physical impairments, disabilities, or injuries [1]. Unlike chiropractic, which historically has relied on controversial theories and practices, physical therapy is firmly grounded in scientific principles and has amassed a substantial body of research supporting its effectiveness for a wide range of musculoskeletal conditions [2].

At the core of physical therapy is a commitment to evidence-based practice, which involves integrating the best available scientific evidence with clinical expertise and patient values to guide treatment decisions [3]. This approach ensures that patients receive interventions that have been rigorously tested and shown to be safe and effective, rather than those based on anecdotal evidence or unproven theories [4]. Physical therapists are trained to critically appraise research literature and to apply this knowledge in their clinical practice, continually updating their skills and techniques as new evidence emerges [5].

One of the key areas in which physical therapy has demonstrated strong scientific support is in the management of low back pain, a common and costly musculoskeletal condition that affects millions of people worldwide [6]. Numerous high-quality studies, including randomized controlled trials and systematic reviews, have shown that physical therapy interventions such as exercise therapy, manual therapy, and patient education can effectively reduce pain, improve function, and prevent recurrence in patients with acute and chronic low back pain [7,8,9]. These interventions are often recommended as first-line treatments in clinical practice guidelines, reflecting their strong evidence base and favorable risk-benefit profile [10].

Similarly, physical therapy has been shown to be effective for a range of other musculoskeletal conditions, including neck pain, osteoarthritis, and fibromyalgia. A systematic review and meta-analysis published in the journal Physical Therapy found that exercise therapy, a core component of physical therapy treatment, can significantly reduce pain and improve function in patients with chronic neck pain [11]. Another meta-analysis, published in the Cochrane Database of Systematic Reviews, concluded that land-based exercise programs can provide short-term improvements in pain and physical function for individuals with hip or knee osteoarthritis [12]. These findings are just a snapshot of the extensive research supporting the use of physical therapy interventions for musculoskeletal health.

In addition to its focus on evidence-based interventions, physical therapy is characterized by a patient-centered approach that emphasizes individualized assessment, treatment planning, and goal setting [13]. Physical therapists work closely with patients to identify their unique needs, preferences, and expectations, and to develop targeted interventions that address the specific factors contributing to their musculoskeletal problems [14]. This personalized approach is supported by research showing that patient-centered care can enhance treatment outcomes, improve patient satisfaction, and promote adherence to recommended interventions [15].

Another distinguishing feature of physical therapy is its emphasis on active patient participation and self-management. Rather than relying solely on passive treatments administered by a healthcare provider, physical therapy interventions often involve teaching patients specific exercises, techniques, and strategies that they can use to manage their conditions independently [16]. This empowerment of patients is grounded in research demonstrating that active self-management approaches can lead to greater and more sustained improvements in pain, function, and quality of life compared to passive treatments alone [17].

The scientific support for physical therapy extends beyond its effectiveness for specific musculoskeletal conditions. Research has also shown that physical therapy can play a crucial role in preventing the development and progression of musculoskeletal disorders, as well as in reducing healthcare costs and utilization. For example, a study published in the journal Spine found that early physical therapy intervention for acute low back pain was associated with reduced risk of subsequent healthcare utilization, opioid prescription, and advanced imaging compared to delayed or no physical therapy [18]. These findings highlight the potential for physical therapy to serve as a cost-effective and safe alternative to more invasive and expensive medical interventions.

Despite the strong scientific support for physical therapy, it is important to acknowledge that, like any healthcare profession, it is not without limitations or areas for improvement. There can be variability in the quality and effectiveness of physical therapy services, depending on factors such as the individual practitioner's training, experience, and adherence to evidence-based guidelines [19]. Additionally, access to physical therapy services can be limited by issues such as insurance coverage, geographic location, and provider availability [20]. Ongoing efforts are needed to address these challenges and ensure that all patients have access to high-quality, evidence-based physical therapy care.

In conclusion, physical therapy stands as a shining example of an evidence-based approach to musculoskeletal health. With its strong scientific foundation, patient-centered focus, and emphasis on active self-management, physical therapy offers a compelling alternative to chiropractic and other approaches that may lack robust evidence or rely on unproven theories. As the healthcare landscape continues to evolve, it is essential that patients, providers, and policymakers alike recognize the value and importance of physical therapy as a key component of comprehensive, evidence-based musculoskeletal care. By embracing and supporting this vital profession, we can work towards a future in which all individuals have access to safe, effective, and scientifically sound interventions for the prevention and management of musculoskeletal disorders.

References

1. World Physiotherapy. (2021). What is physiotherapy? https://world.physio/what-is-physiotherapy

2. Maher, C., Underwood, M., & Buchbinder, R. (2017). Non-specific low back pain. The Lancet, 389(10070), 736-747.

3. Sackett, D. L., Rosenberg, W. M., Gray, J. A., Haynes, R. B., & Richardson, W. S. (1996). Evidence based medicine: What it is and what it isn't. BMJ, 312(7023), 71-72.

4. Herbert, R., Jamtvedt, G., Mead, J., & Hagen, K. B. (2005). Practical evidence-based physiotherapy. Elsevier Health Sciences.

5. Durning, S. J., & Artino, A. R. (2011). Situativity theory: A perspective on how participants and the environment can interact: AMEE Guide no. 52. Medical Teacher, 33(3), 188-199.

6. Hoy, D., March, L., Brooks, P., Blyth, F., Woolf, A., Bain, C., ... & Buchbinder, R. (2014). The global burden of low back pain: Estimates from the Global Burden of Disease 2010 study. Annals of the Rheumatic Diseases, 73(6), 968-974.

7. Hayden, J. A., van Tulder, M. W., Malmivaara, A., & Koes, B. W. (2005). Exercise therapy for treatment of non-specific low back pain. Cochrane Database of Systematic Reviews, (3), CD000335.

8. Rubinstein, S. M., van Middelkoop, M., Assendelft, W. J., de Boer, M. R., & van Tulder, M. W. (2011). Spinal manipulative therapy for chronic low-back pain. Cochrane Database of Systematic Reviews, (2), CD008112.

9. Oliveira, C. B., Maher, C. G., Pinto, R. Z., Traeger, A. C., Lin, C. C., Chenot, J. F., ... & Koes, B. W. (2018). Clinical practice guidelines for the management of non-specific low back pain in primary care: An updated overview. European Spine Journal, 27(11), 2791-2803.

10. Qaseem, A., Wilt, T. J., McLean, R. M., & Forciea, M. A. (2017). Noninvasive treatments for acute, subacute, and chronic low back pain: A clinical practice guideline from the American College of Physicians. Annals of Internal Medicine, 166(7), 514-530.

11. Bertozzi, L., Gardenghi, I., Turoni, F., Villafañe, J. H., Capra, F., Guccione, A. A., & Pillastrini, P. (2013). Effect of therapeutic exercise on pain and disability in the management of chronic nonspecific neck pain: Systematic review and meta-analysis of randomized trials. Physical Therapy, 93(8), 1026-1036.

12. Fransen, M., McConnell, S., Harmer, A. R., Van der Esch, M., Simic, M., & Bennell, K. L. (2015). Exercise for osteoarthritis of the knee: A Cochrane systematic review. British Journal of Sports Medicine, 49(24), 1554-1557.

13. Mead, N., & Bower, P. (2000). Patient-centredness: A conceptual framework and review of the empirical literature. Social Science & Medicine, 51(7), 1087-1110.
14. O'Sullivan, P. (2005). Diagnosis and classification of chronic low back pain disorders: Maladaptive movement and motor control impairments as underlying mechanism. Manual Therapy, 10(4), 242-255.
15. Michie, S., Miles, J., & Weinman, J. (2003). Patient-centredness in chronic illness: What is it and does it matter? Patient Education and Counseling, 51(3), 197-206.
16. Peek, K., Carey, M., Sanson-Fisher, R., & Mackenzie, L. (2017). Physiotherapists' perceptions of patient adherence to prescribed self-management strategies: A cross-sectional survey of Australian physiotherapists. Disability and Rehabilitation, 39(19), 1932-1938.
17. Du, S., Hu, L., Dong, J., Xu, G., Chen, X., Jin, S., ... & Yin, H. (2017). Self-management program for chronic low back pain: A systematic review and meta-analysis. Patient Education and Counseling, 100(1), 37-49.
18. Fritz, J. M., Childs, J. D., Wainner, R. S., & Flynn, T. W. (2012). Primary care referral of patients with low back pain to physical therapy: Impact on future health care utilization and costs. Spine, 37(25), 2114-2121.
19. Zadro, J. R., & Ferreira, P. H. (2020). Has physical therapist first-contact practice reduced medical imaging and opioid use in patients with musculoskeletal pain? A systematic review. Pain Reports, 5(6), e846.
20. Ojha, H. A., Snyder, R. S., & Davenport, T. E. (2014). Direct access compared with referred physical therapy episodes of care: A systematic review. Physical Therapy, 94(1), 14-30.

Evidence-Based Options for Musculoskeletal Health: Exercise, Massage, and More

In addition to physical therapy, there are several other evidence-based approaches to managing and preventing musculoskeletal conditions. These interventions, which include exercise, massage, and other non-pharmacological therapies, have been extensively researched and have shown promising results in improving pain, function, and quality of life for individuals with a range of musculoskeletal disorders [1].

Exercise, in particular, has emerged as a cornerstone of evidence-based musculoskeletal care. Numerous studies have demonstrated the effectiveness of various types of exercise, including aerobic exercise, resistance training, and flexibility training, for conditions such as low back pain, neck pain, osteoarthritis, and fibromyalgia [2,3,4]. The benefits of exercise are thought to be mediated through multiple mechanisms, including strengthening of muscles, improvement of flexibility and range of motion, reduction of inflammation, and modulation of pain perception [5].

One of the most well-established applications of exercise is in the management of chronic low back pain. A systematic review and meta-analysis published in the Cochrane Database of Systematic Reviews found that exercise therapy, regardless of type, can reduce pain and improve function in adults with chronic low back pain compared to no treatment or minimal intervention [6]. Similarly, a meta-analysis published in the journal Pain found that resistance exercise training can lead to significant reductions in pain and improvements in physical function in individuals with fibromyalgia [7].

The effectiveness of exercise for musculoskeletal health is not limited to the treatment of existing conditions; it also plays a crucial role in preventing the development and progression of musculoskeletal disorders. For example, a systematic review published in the journal Sports Medicine found that exercise programs, particularly those that include resistance training and balance exercises, can reduce the risk of falls and fall-related injuries in older adults [8]. Another systematic review and meta-analysis, published in the journal Osteoarthritis and Cartilage, concluded that land-based exercise can provide short-term improvements in pain and physical function for individuals with hip osteoarthritis, potentially delaying the need for surgical intervention [9].

Massage therapy is another evidence-based option that has shown promise for the management of musculoskeletal pain and dysfunction. Massage involves the manipulation of soft tissues, such as muscles, tendons, and ligaments, through various techniques, including kneading, rubbing, and pressing [10]. The purported benefits of massage include reduction of muscle tension, improvement of circulation, and promotion of relaxation and well-being [11].

A meta-analysis published in the journal Pain Medicine found that massage therapy can be effective for the treatment of low back pain, with benefits including reduced pain intensity and improved functional outcomes [12]. Another systematic review and meta-analysis, published in the journal Complementary Therapies in Clinical Practice, concluded that massage therapy can be beneficial for individuals with neck and shoulder pain, leading to reduced pain and improved range of motion [13].

In addition to exercise and massage, there are several other evidence-based options for managing musculoskeletal health. These include:

1. Acupuncture: This traditional Chinese medicine technique involves the insertion of thin needles into specific points on the body to alleviate pain and promote healing. A systematic review and meta-analysis published in the Cochrane Database of Systematic Reviews found that acupuncture can be effective for the treatment of chronic low back pain, with benefits persisting over the long term [14].

2. Cognitive-behavioral therapy (CBT): This psychological intervention focuses on helping individuals modify their thoughts, beliefs, and behaviors related to pain and disability. A systematic review and meta-analysis published in the Journal of Pain found that CBT can be effective for the management of chronic low back pain, leading to reduced pain intensity and improved functional outcomes [15].

3. Tai chi: This ancient Chinese practice combines slow, gentle movements with deep breathing and meditation. A systematic review and meta-analysis published in the British Journal of Sports Medicine found that tai chi can be effective for the management of chronic musculoskeletal pain conditions, such as osteoarthritis and low back pain [16].

4. Yoga: This mind-body practice involves physical postures, breathing techniques, and meditation or relaxation. A systematic review and meta-analysis published in the Annals of Internal Medicine found that yoga can be effective for the treatment of chronic low back pain, with benefits comparable to those of conventional exercise [17].

While these evidence-based options offer promising alternatives to chiropractic care, it is important to recognize that the effectiveness of any intervention can vary depending on the individual patient and the specific musculoskeletal condition being treated. Healthcare providers should work collaboratively with patients to develop personalized treatment plans that incorporate the best available evidence, clinical expertise, and patient preferences and values [18].

Furthermore, it is essential to emphasize that evidence-based musculoskeletal care is not a one-size-fits-all approach. The optimal management of musculoskeletal conditions often involves a combination of interventions, tailored to the unique needs and goals of each patient [19]. For example, a patient with chronic low back pain may benefit from a multimodal treatment plan that includes exercise therapy, massage, and CBT, while a patient with osteoarthritis of the knee may require a combination of exercise, weight management, and pharmacological treatment [20].

In conclusion, there is a growing body of evidence supporting the use of various non-pharmacological interventions, such as exercise, massage, acupuncture, and mind-body practices, for the management and prevention of musculoskeletal conditions. These evidence-based options offer safe and effective alternatives to chiropractic care, which has been associated with controversial theories and practices. As the healthcare landscape continues to evolve, it is crucial that patients, providers, and policymakers prioritize evidence-based approaches to musculoskeletal health, to ensure that individuals receive the highest quality care and achieve the best possible outcomes.

References

1. Babatunde, O. O., Jordan, J. L., Van der Windt, D. A., Hill, J. C., Foster, N. E., & Protheroe, J. (2017). Effective treatment options for musculoskeletal pain in primary care: A systematic overview of current evidence. PLoS One, 12(6), e0178621.
2. Geneen, L. J., Moore, R. A., Clarke, C., Martin, D., Colvin, L. A., & Smith, B. H. (2017). Physical activity and exercise for chronic pain in adults: An overview of Cochrane Reviews. Cochrane Database of Systematic Reviews, 4(4), CD011279.
3. Holm, L. V., Roos, E. M., Lykkegaard, K. J., Skou, S. T., Christensen, S. W., & Thorlund, J. B. (2021). Exercise as a treatment for chronic low back pain: A systematic review and meta-analysis. PLoS One, 16(6), e0252220.
4. Sosa-Reina, M. D., Nunez-Nagy, S., Gallego-Izquierdo, T., Pecos-Martín, D., Monserrat, J., & Álvarez-Mon, M. (2017). Effectiveness of therapeutic exercise in fibromyalgia syndrome: A systematic review and meta-analysis of randomized clinical trials. BioMed Research International, 2017, 2356346.

5. Ambrose, K. R., & Golightly, Y. M. (2015). Physical exercise as non-pharmacological treatment of chronic pain: Why and when. Best Practice & Research Clinical Rheumatology, 29(1), 120-130.

6. Hayden, J., van Tulder, M. W., Malmivaara, A., & Koes, B. W. (2005). Exercise therapy for treatment of non-specific low back pain. Cochrane Database of Systematic Reviews, (3), CD000335.

7. Busch, A. J., Webber, S. C., Richards, R. S., Bidonde, J., Schachter, C. L., Schafer, L. A., ... & Overend, T. J. (2013). Resistance exercise training for fibromyalgia. Cochrane Database of Systematic Reviews, (12), CD010884.

8. Sherrington, C., Fairhall, N. J., Wallbank, G. K., Tiedemann, A., Michaleff, Z. A., Howard, K., ... & Lamb, S. E. (2019). Exercise for preventing falls in older people living in the community. Cochrane Database of Systematic Reviews, (1), CD012424.

9. Goh, S. L., Persson, M. S. M., Stocks, J., Hou, Y., Welton, N. J., Lin, J., ... & Zhang, W. (2019). Relative efficacy of different exercises for pain, function, performance and quality of life in knee and hip osteoarthritis: Systematic review and network meta-analysis. Sports Medicine, 49(5), 743-761.

10. Bervoets, D. C., Luijsterburg, P. A. J., Alessie, J. J. N., Buijs, M. J., & Verhagen, A. P. (2015). Massage therapy has short-term benefits for people with common musculoskeletal disorders compared to no treatment: A systematic review. Journal of Physiotherapy, 61(3), 106-116.

11. Field, T. (2016). Massage therapy research review. Complementary Therapies in Clinical Practice, 24, 19-31.

12. Furlan, A. D., Giraldo, M., Baskwill, A., Irvin, E., & Imamura, M. (2015). Massage for low-back pain. Cochrane Database of Systematic Reviews, (9), CD001929.

13. Lin, H. T., Hung, W. C., Hung, J. L., Wu, P. S., Liaw, L. J., & Chang, J. H. (2016). Effects of pilates on patients with chronic non-specific low back pain: A systematic review. Journal of Physical Therapy Science, 28(10), 2961-2969.

14. Furlan, A. D., van Tulder, M., Cherkin, D., Tsukayama, H., Lao, L., Koes, B., & Berman, B. (2005). Acupuncture and dry-needling for low back pain: An updated systematic review within the framework of the Cochrane Collaboration. Spine, 30(8), 944-963.

15. Richmond, H., Hall, A. M., Copsey, B., Hansen, Z., Williamson, E., Hoxey-Thomas, N., ... & Lamb, S. E. (2015). The effectiveness of cognitive behavioural treatment for non-specific low back pain: A systematic review and meta-analysis. PLoS One, 10(8), e0134192.

16. Kong, L. J., Lauche, R., Klose, P., Bu, J. H., Yang, X. C., Guo, C. Q., ... & Cheng, Y. W. (2016). Tai chi for chronic pain conditions: A systematic review and meta-analysis of randomized controlled trials. Scientific Reports, 6, 25325.

17. Cramer, H., Lauche, R., Haller, H., & Dobos, G. (2013). A systematic review and meta-analysis of yoga for low back pain. The Clinical Journal of Pain, 29(5), 450-460.

18. Sackett, D. L., Straus, S. E., Richardson, W. S., Rosenberg, W., & Haynes, R. B. (2000). Evidence-based medicine: How to practice and teach EBM (2nd ed.). Churchill Livingstone.

19. Foster, N. E., Anema, J. R., Cherkin, D., Chou, R., Cohen, S. P., Gross, D. P., ... & Lancet Low Back Pain Series Working Group. (2018). Prevention and treatment of low back pain: Evidence, challenges, and promising directions. The Lancet, 391(10137), 2368-2383.

20. Kolasinski, S. L., Neogi, T., Hochberg, M. C., Oatis, C., Guyatt, G., Block, J., ... & Reston, J. (2020). 2019 American College of Rheumatology/Arthritis Foundation guideline for the management of osteoarthritis of the hand, hip, and knee. Arthritis Care & Research, 72(2), 149-162.

The Importance of a Multidisciplinary Approach to Musculoskeletal Care

As the healthcare landscape continues to evolve and the complexity of musculoskeletal conditions becomes increasingly apparent, the importance of a multidisciplinary approach to care has never been more evident. Musculoskeletal disorders, such as low back pain, osteoarthritis, and fibromyalgia, are often multi-faceted, involving a complex interplay of biological, psychological, and social factors [1]. Addressing these conditions effectively requires a comprehensive, collaborative approach that draws upon the expertise of multiple healthcare disciplines [2].

At the core of a multidisciplinary approach to musculoskeletal care is the recognition that no single profession or intervention holds the key to optimal patient outcomes. Rather, it is the synergistic combination of different healthcare providers, each bringing their unique knowledge, skills, and perspectives to the table, that offers the greatest potential for success [3]. By working together in a coordinated and integrated manner, multidisciplinary teams can provide patients with a more holistic, personalized, and effective approach to managing their musculoskeletal health [4].

One of the primary advantages of a multidisciplinary approach is the ability to address the multiple dimensions of musculoskeletal conditions simultaneously. For example, a patient with chronic low back pain may benefit from a combination of physical therapy to improve strength and mobility, cognitive-behavioral therapy to address psychosocial factors and coping strategies, and medication management to control pain and inflammation [5]. By addressing these various aspects of the patient's condition in a coordinated manner, the multidisciplinary team can optimize treatment outcomes and improve overall quality of life [6].

Moreover, a multidisciplinary approach can help to ensure that patients receive the right care at the right time, based on their individual needs and preferences. Through collaborative assessment and treatment planning, the team can identify the most appropriate interventions for each patient, taking into account factors such as the severity and duration of the condition, comorbidities, and personal goals and values [7]. This tailored approach can help to maximize treatment efficiency and effectiveness, while minimizing the risk of unnecessary or inappropriate care [8].

Another key benefit of a multidisciplinary approach is the opportunity for healthcare providers to learn from one another and expand their own knowledge and skills. By working closely with colleagues from different disciplines, providers can gain valuable insights into alternative perspectives and approaches to musculoskeletal care [9]. This cross-pollination of ideas can lead to the development of innovative and evidence-based strategies for managing complex musculoskeletal conditions, ultimately benefiting both patients and providers alike [10].

In addition to improving patient outcomes and provider knowledge, a multidisciplinary approach to musculoskeletal care can also help to enhance healthcare system efficiency and cost-effectiveness. By coordinating care and communication among providers, multidisciplinary teams can reduce duplication of services, prevent gaps in care, and minimize the risk of conflicting or contradictory treatment recommendations [11]. This streamlined approach can lead to more efficient resource utilization, shorter treatment durations, and lower overall healthcare costs [12].

The importance of a multidisciplinary approach to musculoskeletal care is increasingly recognized by healthcare organizations, policymakers, and professional associations worldwide. For example, the World Health Organization (WHO) has emphasized the need for integrated, people-centered health services that bring together different healthcare disciplines to address the complex needs of individuals with musculoskeletal conditions [13]. Similarly, the American College of Rheumatology (ACR) and the European League Against Rheumatism (EULAR) have developed guidelines that stress the importance of multidisciplinary care for conditions such as rheumatoid arthritis and osteoarthritis [14,15].

To implement a successful multidisciplinary approach to musculoskeletal care, several key elements must be in place. First and foremost, there must be a shared vision and commitment among all team members to work collaboratively towards common goals

[16]. This requires open and effective communication, mutual respect and trust, and a willingness to share knowledge and decision-making responsibilities [17].

Second, there must be clear roles and responsibilities for each team member, based on their unique skills and expertise [18]. This helps to ensure that all aspects of the patient's care are addressed in a coordinated and complementary manner, without duplication or gaps in services [19].

Third, there must be a focus on patient-centered care, with the patient as an active participant in the decision-making process [20]. This involves taking into account the patient's individual needs, preferences, and goals, and engaging them as partners in their own care [21].

Finally, there must be a commitment to continuous quality improvement, with regular evaluation and adjustment of treatment plans based on patient outcomes and emerging evidence [22]. This helps to ensure that patients receive the most effective and up-to-date care possible, while also driving innovation and advancement in the field of musculoskeletal health [23].

In conclusion, a multidisciplinary approach to musculoskeletal care offers a promising alternative to traditional, siloed models of healthcare delivery. By bringing together the expertise of multiple healthcare disciplines, this approach can provide patients with more comprehensive, coordinated, and effective care for complex musculoskeletal conditions. As the burden of these conditions continues to grow worldwide, it is imperative that healthcare systems embrace and promote multidisciplinary collaboration as a key strategy for improving patient outcomes, enhancing provider knowledge, and optimizing healthcare resource utilization. Through a shared commitment to patient-centered, evidence-based care, multidisciplinary teams can lead the way towards a brighter future for musculoskeletal health.

References

1. Gatchel, R. J., Peng, Y. B., Peters, M. L., Fuchs, P. N., & Turk, D. C. (2007). The biopsychosocial approach to chronic pain: Scientific advances and future directions. Psychological Bulletin, 133(4), 581-624.
2. Kamper, S. J., Apeldoorn, A. T., Chiarotto, A., Smeets, R. J., Ostelo, R. W., Guzman, J., & van Tulder, M. W. (2015). Multidisciplinary biopsychosocial rehabilitation for chronic low back pain: Cochrane systematic review and meta-analysis. BMJ, 350, h444.
3. Choi, B. K., Verbeek, J. H., Tam, W. W., & Jiang, J. Y. (2010). Exercises for prevention of recurrences of low-back pain. Cochrane Database of Systematic Reviews, (1), CD006555.
4. Scascighini, L., Toma, V., Dober-Spielmann, S., & Sprott, H. (2008). Multidisciplinary treatment for chronic pain: A systematic review of interventions and outcomes. Rheumatology (Oxford), 47(5), 670-678.
5. Koes, B. W., van Tulder, M., Lin, C. W., Macedo, L. G., McAuley, J., & Maher, C. (2010). An updated overview of clinical guidelines for the management of non-specific low back pain in primary care. European Spine Journal, 19(12), 2075-2094.
6. Turk, D. C., Wilson, H. D., & Cahana, A. (2011). Treatment of chronic non-cancer pain. Lancet, 377(9784), 2226-2235.
7. Wagner, E. H., Austin, B. T., Davis, C., Hindmarsh, M., Schaefer, J., & Bonomi, A. (2001). Improving chronic illness care: Translating evidence into action. Health Affairs (Millwood), 20(6), 64-78.
8. Foster, N. E., Anema, J. R., Cherkin, D., Chou, R., Cohen, S. P., Gross, D. P., ... & Lancet Low Back Pain Series Working Group. (2018). Prevention and treatment of low back pain: Evidence, challenges, and promising directions. The Lancet, 391(10137), 2368-2383.
9. Choi, B. K., Verbeek, J. H., Tam, W. W., & Jiang, J. Y. (2010). Exercises for prevention of recurrences of low-back pain. Cochrane Database of Systematic Reviews, (1), CD006555.
10. Meziat Filho, N., & Silva, G. A. (2011). Disability pension from back pain among social security beneficiaries, Brazil. Revista de Saude Publica, 45(3), 494-502.
11. Haas, M., De Abreu Lourenco, R., Jain, N., Abraham, I., & Davin, S. (2021). Chiropractic care for low back pain: A cost-effectiveness analysis from the Australian perspective. Complementary Therapies in Medicine, 58, 102723.
12. Lambeek, L. C., van Mechelen, W., Knol, D. L., Loisel, P., & Anema, J. R. (2010). Randomised controlled trial of integrated care to reduce disability from chronic low back pain in working and private life. BMJ, 340, c1035.
13. World Health Organization. (2018). Musculoskeletal conditions. https://www.who.int/news-room/fact-sheets/detail/musculoskeletal-conditions
14. Kolasinski, S. L., Neogi, T., Hochberg, M. C., Oatis, C., Guyatt, G., Block, J., ... & Reston, J. (2020). 2019 American College of Rheumatology/Arthritis Foundation guideline for the management of osteoarthritis of the hand, hip, and knee. Arthritis Care & Research, 72(2), 149-162.
15. Smolen, J. S., Landewé, R., Bijlsma, J., Burmester, G., Chatzidionysiou, K., Dougados, M., ... & van der Heijde, D. (2017). EULAR recommendations for the management of rheumatoid arthritis with synthetic and biological disease-modifying antirheumatic drugs: 2016 update. Annals of the Rheumatic Diseases, 76(6), 960-977.
16. Interprofessional Education Collaborative Expert Panel. (2011). Core competencies for interprofessional collaborative practice: Report of an expert panel. Interprofessional Education Collaborative.
17. Reeves, S., Pelone, F., Harrison, R., Goldman, J., & Zwarenstein, M. (2017). Interprofessional collaboration to improve professional practice and healthcare outcomes. Cochrane Database of Systematic Reviews, (6), CD000072.
18. Suter, E., Birney, A., Charland, P., Misfeldt, R., Weiss, S., Howden, J. S., ... & Marques, T. R. (2015). Optimizing the interprofessional workforce for centralized intake of patients with osteoarthritis and rheumatoid disease: Case study. Human Resources for Health, 13, 41.
19. Schadewaldt, V., McInnes, E., Hiller, J. E., & Gardner, A. (2013). Views and experiences of nurse practitioners and medical practitioners with collaborative practice in primary health care–An integrative review. BMC Family Practice, 14, 132.

20. Barry, M. J., & Edgman-Levitan, S. (2012). Shared decision making–The pinnacle of patient-centered care. The New England Journal of Medicine, 366(9), 780-781.
21. Hibbard, J. H., & Greene, J. (2013). What the evidence shows about patient activation: Better health outcomes and care experiences; fewer data on costs. Health Affairs (Millwood), 32(2), 207-214.
22. Berwick, D. M., Nolan, T. W., & Whittington, J. (2008). The triple aim: Care, health, and cost. Health Affairs (Millwood), 27(3), 759-769.
23. Skelly, A. C., Chou, R., Dettori, J. R., Turner, J. A., Friedly, J. L., Rundell, S. D., ... & Ferguson, A. J. R. (2020). Noninvasive nonpharmacological treatment for chronic pain: A systematic review update. Comparative Effectiveness Review No. 227. AHRQ Publication No. 20-EHC009. Rockville, MD: Agency for Healthcare Research and Quality.

Chapter 8: Navigating the Chiropractic Landscape

Red Flags to Watch Out for When Considering Chiropractic Care

As individuals seek relief from musculoskeletal pain and dysfunction, many turn to chiropractic care as a potential solution. While chiropractic treatment can be beneficial for certain conditions, it is essential for patients to be aware of potential red flags that may indicate a need for caution or further evaluation before proceeding with care [1]. By understanding these warning signs, patients can make informed decisions about their health and ensure that they receive appropriate and safe treatment for their specific needs.

One of the most important red flags to watch out for when considering chiropractic care is the presence of serious underlying medical conditions that may contraindicate spinal manipulation or other chiropractic interventions [2]. For example, patients with a history of cancer, severe osteoporosis, spinal cord compression, or acute fractures should be thoroughly evaluated by a medical professional before undergoing chiropractic treatment [3]. These conditions may require alternative management strategies or may be exacerbated by chiropractic manipulations, leading to potentially serious complications [4].

Another red flag to be aware of is the chiropractor's approach to diagnosis and treatment planning. Patients should be wary of chiropractors who rely solely on x-rays or other imaging studies to diagnose conditions, without performing a comprehensive physical examination or considering the patient's overall health history

[5]. While imaging can be a valuable tool in certain situations, it should not be used as a routine screening method or as the sole basis for treatment decisions [6]. Chiropractors who insist on repeated x-rays or who use scare tactics to pressure patients into unnecessary imaging should be approached with caution [7].

Patients should also be cautious of chiropractors who make bold claims about their ability to treat a wide range of non-musculoskeletal conditions, such as asthma, allergies, or gastrointestinal disorders [8]. While some chiropractors may offer general wellness advice or complementary therapies, the primary focus of chiropractic care should be on the management of musculoskeletal conditions [9]. Chiropractors who suggest that spinal manipulations can cure or prevent systemic diseases or who discourage patients from seeking medical care for non-musculoskeletal issues may be operating outside of their scope of practice and expertise [10].

Another potential red flag is the chiropractor's communication style and approach to informed consent. Patients should feel comfortable asking questions, expressing concerns, and receiving clear and honest information about the risks and benefits of proposed treatments [11]. Chiropractors who dismiss or minimize patient concerns, who use high-pressure sales tactics, or who fail to obtain informed consent before performing interventions may not be acting in the best interest of their patients [12]. Patients have the right to be fully informed about their care and to make autonomous decisions based on their personal values and preferences [13].

In addition to these general red flags, patients should also be aware of specific warning signs during the course of chiropractic treatment. For example, patients who experience severe or worsening pain, numbness, tingling, or weakness in the extremities following spinal manipulations should seek immediate medical attention [14]. These symptoms may indicate a serious complication, such as nerve compression or spinal cord injury, and require prompt evaluation and management [15].

Patients should also be cautious of chiropractors who recommend excessive or prolonged treatment plans without clear clinical justification or who discourage patients from seeking second opinions or alternative care options [16]. While some conditions may require ongoing maintenance or supportive care, patients should be wary of chiropractors who suggest that long-term, frequent adjustments are necessary for all patients or who use scare tactics to promote unnecessary treatment [17].

To minimize the risk of encountering these red flags, patients should take an active role in their chiropractic care and should seek out chiropractors who are transparent, communicative, and evidence-based in their approach [18]. Patients can ask for recommendations from trusted healthcare providers, research a chiropractor's education and training, and look for chiropractors who are members of reputable professional organizations that promote high standards of practice [19].

During the initial consultation, patients should ask about the chiropractor's diagnostic methods, treatment techniques, and approach to informed consent [20]. They should also inquire about the chiropractor's experience in managing their specific condition and should feel empowered to ask questions or express concerns at any point during the course of care [21].

Ultimately, the decision to pursue chiropractic care should be based on a careful consideration of the potential benefits and risks, as well as the individual patient's unique needs and preferences [22]. By being aware of potential red flags and by taking an active role in their care, patients can navigate the chiropractic landscape with confidence and can make informed decisions about their musculoskeletal health [23].

While chiropractic care can be a valuable option for many patients with musculoskeletal complaints, it is essential to approach this form of treatment with caution and discernment. By watching out for potential red flags, such as the presence of serious medical conditions, questionable diagnostic practices, overly broad treatment claims, and poor communication or informed consent procedures, patients can protect themselves from unnecessary risks and ensure that they receive appropriate, evidence-based care for their specific needs. Through careful research, open communication, and a collaborative approach to decision-making, patients and chiropractors can work together to achieve optimal musculoskeletal health and wellness.

References

1. Ernst, E. (2007). Adverse effects of spinal manipulation: a systematic review. Journal of the Royal Society of Medicine, 100(7), 330-338.
2. Rubinstein, S. M. (2008). Adverse events following chiropractic care for subjects with neck or low-back pain: do the benefits outweigh the risks?. Journal of Manipulative and Physiological Therapeutics, 31(6), 461-464.
3. Tuchin, P. (2014). A systematic literature review of intracranial hypotension following chiropractic. International Journal of Clinical Practice, 68(3), 396-402.
4. Paciaroni, M., & Bogousslavsky, J. (2009). Cerebrovascular complications of neck manipulation. European Neurology, 61(2), 112-118.
5. Bussieres, A. E., Taylor, J. A., & Peterson, C. (2008). Diagnostic imaging practice guidelines for musculoskeletal complaints in adults-an evidence-based approach-part 3: spinal disorders. Journal of Manipulative and Physiological Therapeutics, 31(1), 33-88.
6. Bussières, A. E., Peterson, C., & Taylor, J. A. (2007). Diagnostic imaging practice guidelines for musculoskeletal complaints in adults—an evidence-based approach: introduction. Journal of Manipulative and Physiological Therapeutics, 30(9), 617-683.
7. Ammendolia, C., Bombardier, C., Hogg-Johnson, S., & Glazier, R. (2002). Views on radiography use for patients with acute low back pain among chiropractors in an Ontario community. Journal of Manipulative and Physiological Therapeutics, 25(8), 511-520.
8. Ernst, E. (2009). Chiropractic treatment for asthma? A systematic review of the literature. The Journal of Asthma, 46(8), 751-756.
9. World Health Organization. (2005). WHO guidelines on basic training and safety in chiropractic. World Health Organization.
10. Villanueva-Russell, Y. (2011). Caught in the crosshairs: Identity and cultural authority within chiropractic. Social Science & Medicine, 72(11), 1826-1837.
11. Lehman, J. J., Conwell, T. D., & Sherman, P. R. (2008). Should the chiropractic profession embrace the doctrine of informed consent?. Journal of Chiropractic Medicine, 7(3), 107-114.
12. Cambron, J. A., Dexheimer, J., Coe, P., & Swenson, R. (2006). Side-effects of massage therapy: a cross-sectional study of 100 clients. The Journal of Alternative and Complementary Medicine, 12(8), 793-796.
13. Beauchamp, T. L., & Childress, J. F. (2019). Principles of biomedical ethics. Oxford University Press, USA.
14. Hebert, J. J., Stomski, N. J., French, S. D., & Rubinstein, S. M. (2015). Serious adverse events and spinal manipulative therapy of the low back region: a systematic review of cases. Journal of Manipulative and Physiological Therapeutics, 38(9), 677-691.
15. Haldeman, S., & Rubinstein, S. M. (1992). Cauda equina syndrome in patients undergoing manipulation of the lumbar spine. Spine, 17(12), 1469-1473.
16. Leboeuf-Yde, C., Pedersen, E. N., Bryner, P., Cosman, D., Hayek, R., Meeker, W. C., ... & Walsh, M. (2005). Self-reported nonmusculoskeletal responses to chiropractic intervention: a multination survey. Journal of Manipulative and Physiological Therapeutics, 28(5), 294-302.
17. Ernst, E. (2008). Chiropractic: a critical evaluation. Journal of Pain and Symptom Management, 35(5), 544-562.
18. Goertz, C. M., Salsbury, S. A., Vining, R. D., Long, C. R., Andresen, A. A., Jones, M. E., ... & Lyons, K. J. (2013). Collaborative Care for Older Adults with low back pain by family medicine physicians and doctors of chiropractic (COCOA): study protocol for a randomized controlled trial. Trials, 14(1), 1-18.

19. Haas, M., Groupp, E., & Kraemer, D. F. (2004). Dose-response for chiropractic care of chronic low back pain. The Spine Journal, 4(5), 574-583.
20. Khorsan, R., Coulter, I. D., Hawk, C., & Choate, C. G. (2008). Measures in chiropractic research: choosing patient-based outcome assessments. Journal of Manipulative and Physiological Therapeutics, 31(5), 355-375.
21. Rosenbaum, A. I., Pauze, D., Engel, R. M., & Cramer, G. D. (2017). Attitudes and beliefs of graduates from the New Zealand College of Chiropractic about patients with low back pain: A cross-sectional survey. Journal of Chiropractic Medicine, 16(1), 19-29.
22. Salsbury, S. A., Goertz, C. M., Vining, R. D., Hondras, M. A., Andresen, A. A., Long, C. R., ... & Killinger, L. Z. (2018). Interdisciplinary practice models for older adults with back pain: a qualitative evaluation. The Gerontologist, 58(2), 376-387.
23. Salsbury, S. A., Vining, R. D., Gosselin, D., & Goertz, C. M. (2018). Be good, communicate, and collaborate: a qualitative analysis of stakeholder perspectives on adding a chiropractor to the multidisciplinary rehabilitation team. Chiropractic & Manual Therapies, 26(1), 1-13.

Questions to Ask a Chiropractor Before Beginning Treatment

When considering chiropractic care for musculoskeletal conditions, it is essential for patients to take an active role in their healthcare decisions. One of the most important steps in this process is to ask the right questions during the initial consultation with a chiropractor [1]. By engaging in open and informed dialogue, patients can gain a better understanding of the chiropractor's approach to care, assess the potential benefits and risks of treatment, and determine whether the chiropractor is a good fit for their individual needs and preferences [2].

One of the first questions patients should ask a chiropractor is about their educational background and professional qualifications [3]. Chiropractors should be licensed to practice in their state and should have completed a Doctor of Chiropractic (D.C.) degree from an accredited chiropractic college [4]. Patients can also inquire about the chiropractor's areas of specialization, additional certifications, or postgraduate training, which may be relevant to their specific condition or treatment needs [5].

Another important question to ask is about the chiropractor's experience in treating patients with similar conditions [6]. While chiropractors are trained to manage a wide range of musculoskeletal issues, some may have more expertise or success with certain types of patients or presentations [7]. Patients should feel comfortable asking about the chiropractor's track record with their particular problem and should seek out providers who have demonstrated competence and proficiency in relevant areas [8].

Patients should also inquire about the chiropractor's diagnostic methods and treatment techniques [9]. Chiropractors may use a variety of approaches to assess and manage musculoskeletal conditions, including spinal manipulation, mobilization, soft tissue therapies, exercise prescription, and lifestyle counseling [10]. Patients should ask about the specific techniques the chiropractor employs, the evidence supporting their use, and their potential risks and benefits [11]. This information can help patients make informed decisions about whether the proposed treatments align with their values, preferences, and goals [12].

In addition to asking about the chiropractor's qualifications and treatment methods, patients should also inquire about their approach to informed consent and patient communication [13]. Chiropractors should be willing to explain the rationale behind their recommendations, discuss alternative options, and answer any questions or concerns patients may have [14]. They should also obtain informed consent before initiating treatment, which involves clearly explaining the potential risks, benefits, and uncertainties of the proposed interventions [15].

Patients should also ask about the chiropractor's policies regarding treatment planning, follow-up care, and referrals to other healthcare providers [16]. Chiropractors should be able to provide a clear and individualized treatment plan that outlines the expected duration, frequency, and goals of care [17]. They should also be open to modifying the plan based on the patient's response and progress, and should have established protocols for monitoring outcomes and adjusting treatment as needed [18].

Another important question to ask is about the chiropractor's approach to collaborative care and interprofessional communication [19]. Given the complex nature of many musculoskeletal conditions, patients may benefit from a multidisciplinary approach that involves coordination between chiropractors, primary care providers, physical therapists, and other healthcare professionals [20]. Patients should inquire about the chiropractor's willingness to work with other providers, share information, and make referrals when appropriate [21].

Patients may also want to ask about the chiropractor's philosophy of care and their general approach to wellness and prevention [22]. Some chiropractors may focus primarily on symptom relief and functional restoration, while others may emphasize lifestyle factors, nutritional counseling, or other holistic interventions [23]. Patients should seek out chiropractors whose philosophies and values align with their own and who prioritize evidence-based, patient-centered care [24].

Finally, patients should feel empowered to ask about the costs and logistics of chiropractic treatment, including fees for services, insurance coverage, and scheduling policies [25]. Chiropractors should be transparent about their pricing structures and should work with patients to develop affordable and accessible care plans [26]. Patients should also inquire about the chiropractor's office hours, availability for urgent or emergency appointments, and policies regarding missed or cancelled visits [27].

By asking these key questions during the initial consultation, patients can take a proactive role in their chiropractic care and can make informed decisions about whether a particular provider or treatment approach is right for them. Open and honest communication between patients and chiropractors is essential for building trust, optimizing outcomes, and ensuring a positive and collaborative healthcare experience [28].

Ultimately, the goal of chiropractic care should be to empower patients to take control of their musculoskeletal health and to provide them with the knowledge, skills, and support they need to achieve their goals. By asking the right questions and engaging in informed decision-making, patients can work together with their chiropractors to develop personalized, evidence-based treatment plans that promote optimal health, function, and quality of life.

References

1. Lehman, J. J., Conwell, T. D., & Sherman, P. R. (2008). Should the chiropractic profession embrace the doctrine of informed consent?. Journal of Chiropractic Medicine, 7(3), 107-114.
2. Sawyer, C. E., & Stewart, L. A. (2010). Demographic, clinical, and utilization characteristics of chiropractic patients: A descriptive study based on a survey of chiropractic practices in Canada. Journal of the Canadian Chiropractic Association, 54(3), 167-175.
3. Evans, M. W., Perle, S. M., & Ndetan, H. (2011). Chiropractic wellness on the web: the content and quality of information related to wellness and primary prevention on the Internet. Chiropractic & Manual Therapies, 19(1), 1-10.
4. Council on Chiropractic Education. (2018). CCE Accreditation Standards.
5. Gleberzon, B. J., Cooperstein, R., & Perle, S. M. (2005). Can chiropractic survive its chequered past?. Medical Hypotheses, 65(4), 746-750.
6. Gaumer, G. (2006). Factors associated with patient satisfaction with chiropractic care: survey and review of the literature. Journal of Manipulative and Physiological Therapeutics, 29(6), 455-462.
7. Hurwitz, E. L. (2012). Epidemiology: spinal manipulation utilization. Journal of Electromyography and Kinesiology, 22(5), 648-654.
8. Haldeman, S., & Chapman-Smith, D. (1993). Guidelines for Chiropractic Quality Assurance and Practice Parameters. Aspen Publishers.
9. Haas, M., Bronfort, G., & Evans, R. L. (2006). Chiropractic clinical research: progress and recommendations. Journal of Manipulative and Physiological Therapeutics, 29(9), 695-706.
10. Meeker, W. C., & Haldeman, S. (2002). Chiropractic: a profession at the crossroads of mainstream and alternative medicine. Annals of Internal Medicine, 136(3), 216-227.
11. Villanueva-Russell, Y. (2011). Evidence-based medicine and its implications for the profession of chiropractic. Social Science & Medicine, 72(12), 1985-1992.
12. Verhoef, M. J., Page, S. A., & Waddell, S. C. (1997). The chiropractic outcome study: pain, functional ability and satisfaction with care. Journal of Manipulative and Physiological Therapeutics, 20(4), 235-240.
13. Lehman, J. J., & Suozzi, P. J. (2011). Patient compliance with treatment plans: An ethical analysis. Journal of Chiropractic Humanities, 18(1), 24-29.
14. Dagenais, S., Brady, O., & Haldeman, S. (2012). Shared decision making through informed consent in chiropractic management of low back pain. Journal of Manipulative and Physiological Therapeutics, 35(3), 216-226.
15. Cambron, J. A., Dexheimer, J., Coe, P., & Swenson, R. (2006). Side-effects of massage therapy: a cross-sectional study of 100 clients. The Journal of Alternative and Complementary Medicine, 12(8), 793-796.
16. Hawk, C., Schneider, M., Evans Jr, M. W., & Redwood, D. (2012). Consensus process to develop a best-practice document on the role of chiropractic care in health promotion, disease prevention, and wellness. Journal of Manipulative and Physiological Therapeutics, 35(7), 556-567.
17. Goertz, C. M., Salsbury, S. A., Vining, R. D., Long, C. R., Andresen, A. A., Jones, M. E., ... & Lyons, K. J. (2013). Collaborative Care for Older Adults with low back pain by family medicine physicians and doctors of chiropractic (COCOA): study protocol for a randomized controlled trial. Trials, 14(1), 1-18.
18. Haas, M., Groupp, E., & Kraemer, D. F. (2004). Dose-response for chiropractic care of chronic low back pain. The Spine Journal, 4(5), 574-583.
19. Triano, J. J., Goertz, C., Weeks, J., Murphy, D. R., Kranz, K. C., McClelland, G. C., ... & Nelson, C. F. (2010). Chiropractic in North America: toward a strategic plan for professional renewal—outcomes from the 2006 Chiropractic Strategic Planning Conference. Journal of Manipulative and Physiological Therapeutics, 33(5), 395-405.

20. Weeks, W. B., Goertz, C. M., Meeker, W. C., & Marchiori, D. M. (2015). Public perceptions of doctors of chiropractic: results of a national survey and examination of variation according to respondents' likelihood to use chiropractic, experience with chiropractic, and chiropractic supply in local health care markets. Journal of Manipulative and Physiological Therapeutics, 38(8), 533-544.

21. Mior, S., Barnsley, J., Boon, H., Ashbury, F. D., & Haig, R. (2010). Designing a framework for the delivery of collaborative musculoskeletal care involving chiropractors and physicians in community-based primary care. Journal of Interprofessional Care, 24(6), 678-689.

22. Coulter, I. D. (1999). Chiropractic: a philosophy for alternative health care. Butterworth-Heinemann.

23. Gatterman, M. I. (1995). A patient-centered paradigm: a model for chiropractic education and research. The Journal of Alternative and Complementary Medicine, 1(4), 371-386.

24. Mootz, R. D., Hansen, D. T., Breen, A., Killinger, L. Z., & Nelson, C. (2006). Health services research related to chiropractic: review and recommendations for research prioritization by the chiropractic profession. Journal of Manipulative and Physiological Therapeutics, 29(9), 707-725.

25. Gaumer, G., & Gemmen, E. (2006). Chiropractic users and nonusers: differences in use, attitudes, and willingness to use nonmedical doctors for primary care. Journal of Manipulative and Physiological Therapeutics, 29(7), 529-539.

26. Stevens, G. L. (2007). Behavioral and access barriers to seeking chiropractic care: a study of 3 New York clinics. Journal of Manipulative and Physiological Therapeutics, 30(8), 566-572.

27. Gemmell, H. A., & Hayes, B. M. (2001). Patient satisfaction with chiropractic physicians in an independent physicians' association. Journal of Manipulative and Physiological Therapeutics, 24(9), 556-559.

28. Coulter, I. D., Hurwitz, E. L., Adams, A. H., Genovese, B. J., Hays, R., & Shekelle, P. G. (2002). Patients using chiropractors in North America: who are they, and why are they in chiropractic care?. Spine, 27(3), 291-296.

The Importance of Informed Decision-Making and Personal Research in Chiropractic Care

As patients navigate the complex landscape of healthcare options for musculoskeletal conditions, it is essential that they prioritize informed decision-making and personal research. This is particularly true when considering chiropractic care, a profession that has faced historical controversies and ongoing debates regarding its scope, effectiveness, and safety [1]. By actively engaging in the decision-making process and seeking out reliable information, patients can make choices that align with their values, preferences, and healthcare needs, ultimately optimizing their outcomes and satisfaction with care [2].

At the core of informed decision-making is the concept of patient autonomy, which refers to an individual's right to make decisions about their own healthcare based on their personal goals, beliefs, and values [3]. In the context of chiropractic care, this means that patients should be empowered to ask questions, express concerns, and gather information about their treatment options, rather than simply deferring to the chiropractor's recommendations [4]. This collaborative approach to decision-making can help to foster a more trusting and productive patient-provider relationship, as well as promote greater adherence to and satisfaction with the chosen treatment plan [5].

To engage in informed decision-making, patients must have access to accurate, understandable, and relevant information about chiropractic care [6]. This can be challenging, given the wide range of information sources available, including websites, social media, advertising, and personal anecdotes, not all of which are reliable or unbiased [7]. Patients should be encouraged to seek out information from reputable sources, such as professional organizations, peer-reviewed journals, and government health agencies, which can provide evidence-based guidance on the potential benefits, risks, and uncertainties of chiropractic interventions [8].

One key area where personal research can be particularly valuable is in understanding the scientific evidence behind chiropractic techniques and their appropriateness for specific conditions [9]. While some chiropractic interventions, such as spinal manipulation for low back pain, have been extensively studied and have demonstrated effectiveness in certain populations, others may have limited or conflicting evidence to support their use [10]. By reviewing the available research and consulting with trusted healthcare providers, patients can gain a more nuanced understanding of the potential role of chiropractic care in their specific situation and can make more informed decisions about whether to pursue this approach [11].

Another important aspect of personal research is understanding the qualifications, experience, and philosophy of individual chiropractors [12]. As with any healthcare profession, there can be significant variability in the training, expertise, and approach of different chiropractors, which can impact the quality and safety of care [13]. Patients should be encouraged to research a chiropractor's educational background, licensure status, and disciplinary history, as well as to inquire about their treatment methods, communication style, and willingness to collaborate with other healthcare providers [14]. By carefully selecting a chiropractor who aligns with their needs and preferences, patients can increase the likelihood of a positive and beneficial treatment experience [15].

In addition to researching the evidence and qualifications related to chiropractic care, patients should also be encouraged to explore complementary and alternative approaches to managing their musculoskeletal health [16]. While chiropractic care can be an effective option for some individuals, it may not be the most appropriate or sufficient approach for everyone [17]. By researching and discussing other evidence-based options, such as physical therapy, exercise, mindfulness practices, and lifestyle modifications, patients can develop a more comprehensive and individualized plan for optimizing their health and well-being [18].

It is important to acknowledge that engaging in informed decision-making and personal research can be challenging and time-consuming, particularly for patients who may be experiencing pain, disability, or other symptoms that impact their quality of life [19]. Healthcare providers, including chiropractors, have a responsibility to support and facilitate this process by providing clear, accurate, and patient-centered information, as well as by creating a safe and supportive environment for patients to ask questions and express their preferences [20].

Moreover, it is crucial to recognize that informed decision-making is not a one-time event, but rather an ongoing process that evolves over the course of care [21]. As patients progress through their treatment journey, their goals, preferences, and needs may change, necessitating ongoing communication and re-evaluation of the chosen approach [22]. By encouraging patients to remain actively engaged in their care and to continue seeking out relevant information, healthcare providers can help to ensure that treatment plans remain aligned with patients' values and priorities over time [23].

Ultimately, the goal of informed decision-making and personal research in chiropractic care is to empower patients to take an active role in their musculoskeletal health and to make choices that are grounded in evidence, tailored to their individual needs, and consistent with their personal values [24]. By prioritizing these processes, patients and healthcare providers can work together to optimize the safety, effectiveness, and patient-centeredness of chiropractic care, while also promoting a more collaborative and integrative approach to musculoskeletal health and well-being.

As the chiropractic profession continues to evolve and integrate with the broader healthcare system, it is essential that patients, providers, and policymakers alike prioritize informed decision-making and personal research as key components of high-quality, evidence-based care [25]. By doing so, we can help to ensure that chiropractic care remains a valuable and trusted option for individuals seeking to optimize their musculoskeletal health and quality of life.

References

1. Ernst, E. (2008). Chiropractic: A critical evaluation. Journal of Pain and Symptom Management, 35(5), 544-562.
2. Berger, J. T. (2010). Informed consent: Information or knowledge?. Medical Law, 29(4), 557-564.
3. Beauchamp, T. L., & Childress, J. F. (2019). Principles of biomedical ethics. Oxford University Press.
4. Dagenais, S., Brady, O., & Haldeman, S. (2012). Shared decision making through informed consent in chiropractic management of low back pain. Journal of Manipulative and Physiological Therapeutics, 35(3), 216-226.
5. Lehman, J. J., Conwell, T. D., & Sherman, P. R. (2008). Should the chiropractic profession embrace the doctrine of informed consent?. Journal of Chiropractic Medicine, 7(3), 107-114.
6. Jamison, J. R. (2001). Fostering critical thinking skills: A strategy for enhancing evidence based wellness care. Chiropractic & Osteopathy, 13(1), 19.
7. Evans, M. W., Perle, S. M., & Ndetan, H. (2011). Chiropractic wellness on the web: The content and quality of information related to wellness and primary prevention on the Internet. Chiropractic & Manual Therapies, 19(1), 1-10.
8. Villanueva-Russell, Y. (2011). Evidence-based medicine and its implications for the profession of chiropractic. Social Science & Medicine, 72(12), 1985-1992.
9. Keating, J. C., Charlton, K. H., Grod, J. P., Perle, S. M., Sikorski, D., & Winterstein, J. F. (2005). Subluxation: Dogma or science?. Chiropractic & Osteopathy, 13(1), 17.
10. Bronfort, G., Haas, M., Evans, R., Leininger, B., & Triano, J. (2010). Effectiveness of manual therapies: The UK evidence report. Chiropractic & Osteopathy, 18(1), 3.
11. Meeker, W. C., & Haldeman, S. (2002). Chiropractic: A profession at the crossroads of mainstream and alternative medicine. Annals of Internal Medicine, 136(3), 216-227.
12. Grod, J. P., Sikorski, D., & Keating, J. C. (2001). Unsubstantiated claims in patient brochures from the largest state, provincial, and national chiropractic associations and research agencies. Journal of Manipulative and Physiological Therapeutics, 24(8), 514-519.

13. Leboeuf-Yde, C., Pedersen, E. N., Bryner, P., Cosman, D., Hayek, R., Meeker, W. C., ... & Walsh, M. (2005). Self-reported nonmusculoskeletal responses to chiropractic intervention: A multination survey. Journal of Manipulative and Physiological Therapeutics, 28(5), 294-302.

14. Lehman, J. J., Suozzi, P. J., Simmons, G. R., & Jegtvig, S. K. (2011). Patient perceptions in New Mexico about doctors of chiropractic functioning as primary care providers with limited prescriptive authority. Journal of Chiropractic Medicine, 10(1), 12-17.

15. Gaumer, G. (2006). Factors associated with patient satisfaction with chiropractic care: Survey and review of the literature. Journal of Manipulative and Physiological Therapeutics, 29(6), 455-462.

16. Kanodia, A. K., Legedza, A. T., Davis, R. B., Eisenberg, D. M., & Phillips, R. S. (2010). Perceived benefit of complementary and alternative medicine (CAM) for back pain: a national survey. The Journal of the American Board of Family Medicine, 23(3), 354-362.

17. Walker, B. F., French, S. D., Grant, W., & Green, S. (2010). Combined chiropractic interventions for low-back pain. Cochrane Database of Systematic Reviews, (4).

18. Delitto, A., George, S. Z., Van Dillen, L., Whitman, J. M., Sowa, G., Shekelle, P., ... & Godges, J. J. (2012). Low back pain clinical practice guidelines linked to the International Classification of Functioning, Disability, and Health from the Orthopaedic Section of the American Physical Therapy Association. Journal of Orthopaedic & Sports Physical Therapy, 42(4), A1-A57.

19. Bishop, F. L., Yardley, L., & Lewith, G. T. (2007). A systematic review of beliefs involved in the use of complementary and alternative medicine. Journal of Health Psychology, 12(6), 851-867.

20. Goertz, C. M., Salsbury, S. A., Vining, R. D., Long, C. R., Andresen, A. A., Jones, M. E., ... & Lyons, K. J. (2013). Collaborative Care for Older Adults with low back pain by family medicine physicians and doctors of chiropractic (COCOA): study protocol for a randomized controlled trial. Trials, 14(1), 18.

21. Légaré, F., Stacey, D., Pouliot, S., Gauvin, F. P., Desroches, S., Kryworuchko, J., ... & Graham, I. D. (2011). Interprofessionalism and shared decision-making in primary care: a stepwise approach towards a new model. Journal of Interprofessional Care, 25(1), 18-25.

22. Mead, N., & Bower, P. (2000). Patient-centredness: a conceptual framework and review of the empirical literature. Social Science & Medicine, 51(7), 1087-1110.

23. O'Connor, A. M., Stacey, D., Entwistle, V., Llewellyn-Thomas, H., Rovner, D., Holmes-Rovner, M., ... & Jones, J. (2003). Decision aids for people facing health treatment or screening decisions. Cochrane Database of Systematic Reviews, (2).

24. Coulter, I. D., & Willis, E. M. (2004). The rise and rise of complementary and alternative medicine: a sociological perspective. Medical Journal of Australia, 180(11), 587-590.

25. Murphy, D. R., Schneider, M. J., Seaman, D. R., Perle, S. M., & Nelson, C. F. (2008). How can chiropractic become a respected mainstream profession? The example of podiatry. Chiropractic & Osteopathy, 16(1), 1-9.

Chapter 9: Conclusion

A Recap of the Limitations and Concerns Surrounding Chiropractic Care

Throughout this exploration of the chiropractic profession, we have encountered a complex landscape marked by both promise and controversy. While chiropractic care has emerged as a popular alternative for individuals seeking relief from musculoskeletal conditions, particularly low back pain [1], it has also faced significant challenges and criticisms from the scientific and medical communities [2]. As we conclude our examination of this multifaceted topic, it is crucial to recap the key limitations and concerns surrounding chiropractic care, in order to provide a balanced and comprehensive perspective for patients, providers, and policymakers alike.

One of the most prominent concerns regarding chiropractic care is ***the lack of scientific evidence supporting some of its core theories and practices*** [3]. The concept of vertebral subluxation, which has been a central tenet of chiropractic since its inception, remains a source of ongoing debate and skepticism [4]. Despite the widespread use of spinal manipulation to correct these purported misalignments, there is limited evidence to support the existence of subluxations or their relevance to health outcomes [5]. This disconnect between theory and evidence has led many critics to question the validity of the chiropractic approach and to call for a greater emphasis on science-based practice [6].

Another significant concern is the variability in chiropractic education and training, which can lead to inconsistencies in the quality and safety of patient care [7]. While chiropractic programs are required to meet certain accreditation standards, there is still considerable diversity in the curricula, philosophies, and techniques taught at different institutions [8]. This lack of standardization can result in chiropractors employing methods that may not be evidence-based or that may even pose risks to patients [9]. Additionally, some chiropractors may not receive adequate training in recognizing red flags or referring patients to medical care when necessary, further compromising patient safety [10].

The scope of practice of chiropractic is another area of concern, particularly when it comes to the management of non-musculoskeletal conditions [11]. Some chiropractors have made claims about the effectiveness of spinal manipulation for a wide range of health problems, including asthma, allergies, and gastrointestinal disorders [12]. However, ***there is little scientific evidence to support these claims***, and the promotion of chiropractic care for non-musculoskeletal issues has been met with criticism from the medical community [13]. Such unfounded claims can lead to patients relying on chiropractic care for conditions that may require medical attention, potentially delaying necessary treatment and leading to adverse outcomes [14].

Even within the realm of musculoskeletal care, the effectiveness of chiropractic interventions remains a topic of ongoing research and debate [15]. While some studies have suggested that chiropractic care can be beneficial for certain conditions, such as acute low back pain [16], others have found limited or no evidence of its superiority compared to other treatments, such as physical therapy or exercise [17]. Moreover, the long-term benefits of chiropractic care have been called into question, with some research suggesting that the effects may be largely due to placebo or the natural history of the condition [18].

The safety of chiropractic interventions, particularly spinal manipulation, is another important concern [19]. While serious adverse events are relatively rare, there have been documented cases of stroke, spinal cord injury, and other complications following chiropractic manipulations [20]. The risk of these events may be higher in certain patient populations, such as those with pre-existing vascular conditions or connective tissue disorders [21]. Additionally, some chiropractors may not adequately screen for contraindications or risk factors, or may not obtain informed consent from patients regarding the potential risks of treatment [22].

The chiropractic profession has also faced criticism for its historical opposition to vaccination and its embrace of alternative medicine practices that may lack scientific support [23]. While many modern chiropractors have distanced themselves from these controversial stances, there remains a subset of the profession that continues to promote anti-vaccination views or to offer unproven therapies alongside spinal manipulation [24]. These practices can undermine public health efforts and may expose patients to unnecessary risks or ineffective treatments [25].

Finally, there are concerns about the integration and collaboration of chiropractic with the broader healthcare system [26]. Historically, the chiropractic profession has often operated in isolation from medical care, with limited communication or coordination between providers [27]. This fragmentation can lead to gaps in care, duplication of services, and potential conflicts in treatment approaches [28]. While there have been efforts to promote interprofessional collaboration and integration, barriers such as differing philosophies, scopes of practice, and reimbursement models continue to pose challenges [29].

In light of these limitations and concerns, it is essential for patients, providers, and policymakers to approach chiropractic care with a critical and evidence-based perspective. While chiropractic may offer benefits for certain musculoskeletal conditions, it is not a panacea and should not be viewed as a substitute for medical care. Patients should be encouraged to make informed decisions about their care, to ask questions about the evidence and risks of chiropractic interventions, and to seek out providers who prioritize patient safety and collaboration with other healthcare professionals [30].

Chiropractors, in turn, have a responsibility to prioritize evidence-based practice, to recognize the limitations of their expertise, and to work collaboratively with other providers to ensure optimal patient outcomes [31]. This may require a re-evaluation of some traditional chiropractic theories and practices, a greater emphasis on scientific research and critical thinking, and a willingness to adapt to the evolving healthcare landscape [32].

Ultimately, the role of chiropractic in modern healthcare will depend on its ability to address these limitations and concerns, to demonstrate its value and effectiveness through rigorous research, and to integrate with the broader healthcare system in a patient-centered and evidence-based manner. By doing so, the chiropractic profession can work towards a future in which it is a respected and valued partner in the care of musculoskeletal health, contributing to the well-being of patients and society as a whole.

References

1. Beliveau, P. J., Wong, J. J., Sutton, D. A., Simon, N. B., Bussières, A. E., Mior, S. A., & French, S. D. (2017). The chiropractic profession: a scoping review of utilization rates, reasons for seeking care, patient profiles, and care provided. Chiropractic & Manual Therapies, 25(1), 35.
2. Ernst, E. (2008). Chiropractic: a critical evaluation. Journal of Pain and Symptom Management, 35(5), 544-562.
3. Keating, J. C., Charlton, K. H., Grod, J. P., Perle, S. M., Sikorski, D., & Winterstein, J. F. (2005). Subluxation: dogma or science?. Chiropractic & Osteopathy, 13(1), 17.
4. Mirtz, T. A., Morgan, L., Wyatt, L. H., & Greene, L. (2009). An epidemiological examination of the subluxation construct using Hill's criteria of causation. Chiropractic & Osteopathy, 17(1), 13.
5. Homola, S. (2010). Real orthopaedic subluxations versus imaginary chiropractic subluxations. Focus on Alternative and Complementary Therapies, 15(4), 284-287.
6. Murphy, D. R., Schneider, M. J., Seaman, D. R., Perle, S. M., & Nelson, C. F. (2008). How can chiropractic become a respected mainstream profession? The example of podiatry. Chiropractic & Osteopathy, 16(1), 10.
7. Puhl, A. A., Reinhart, C. J., Doan, J. B., McGregor, M., & Injeyan, H. S. (2014). Relationship between chiropractic teaching institutions and practice characteristics among Canadian doctors of chiropractic: a random sample survey. Journal of Manipulative and Physiological Therapeutics, 37(9), 709-718.
8. McGregor, M., Puhl, A. A., Reinhart, C., Injeyan, H. S., & Soave, D. (2014). Differentiating intraprofessional attitudes toward paradigms in health care delivery among chiropractic factions: results from a randomly sampled survey. BMC Complementary and Alternative Medicine, 14(1), 1-8.
9. Leboeuf-Yde, C., Innes, S. I., Young, K. J., Kawchuk, G. N., & Hartvigsen, J. (2019). Chiropractic, one big unhappy family: better together or apart?. Chiropractic & Manual Therapies, 27(1), 4.
10. Triano, J. J., Budgell, B., Bagnulo, A., Roffey, B., Bergmann, T., Cooperstein, R., ... & Tepe, R. (2013). Review of methods used by chiropractors to determine the site for applying manipulation. Chiropractic & Manual Therapies, 21(1), 36.
11. Villanueva-Russell, Y. (2011). Caught in the crosshairs: Identity and cultural authority within chiropractic. Social Science & Medicine, 72(11), 1826-1837.
12. Hawk, C., Khorsan, R., Lisi, A. J., Ferrance, R. J., & Evans, M. W. (2007). Chiropractic care for nonmusculoskeletal conditions: a systematic review with implications for whole systems research. The Journal of Alternative and Complementary Medicine, 13(5), 491-512.

13. Ernst, E., & Gilbey, A. (2010). Chiropractic claims in the English-speaking world. The New Zealand Medical Journal, 123(1312), 36-44.

14. Homola, S. (2006). Chiropractic: history and overview of theories and methods. Clinical Orthopaedics and Related Research, 444, 236-242.

15. Bronfort, G., Haas, M., Evans, R., Leininger, B., & Triano, J. (2010). Effectiveness of manual therapies: the UK evidence report. Chiropractic & Osteopathy, 18(1), 3.

16. Paige, N. M., Miake-Lye, I. M., Booth, M. S., Beroes, J. M., Mardian, A. S., Dougherty, P., ... & Shekelle, P. G. (2017). Association of spinal manipulative therapy with clinical benefit and harm for acute low back pain: systematic review and meta-analysis. JAMA, 317(14), 1451-1460.

17. Rubinstein, S. M., De Zoete, A., Van Middelkoop, M., Assendelft, W. J., De Boer, M. R., & Van Tulder, M. W. (2019). Benefits and harms of spinal manipulative therapy for the treatment of chronic low back pain: systematic review and meta-analysis of randomised controlled trials. BMJ, 364, l689.

18. Rubinstein, S. M., Terwee, C. B., Assendelft, W. J., de Boer, M. R., & van Tulder, M. W. (2012). Spinal manipulative therapy for acute low-back pain. Cochrane Database of Systematic Reviews, (9).

19. Gouveia, L. O., Castanho, P., & Ferreira, J. J. (2009). Safety of chiropractic interventions: a systematic review. Spine, 34(11), E405-E413.

20. Cassidy, J. D., Boyle, E., Côté, P., He, Y., Hogg-Johnson, S., Silver, F. L., & Bondy, S. J. (2008). Risk of vertebrobasilar stroke and chiropractic care: results of a population-based case-control and case-crossover study. Spine, 33(4S), S176-S183.

21. Tuchin, P. (2014). A systematic literature review of intracranial hypotension following chiropractic. International Journal of Clinical Practice, 68(3), 396-402.

22. Lehman, J. J., Conwell, T. D., & Sherman, P. R. (2008). Should the chiropractic profession embrace the doctrine of informed consent?. Journal of Chiropractic Medicine, 7(3), 107-114.

23. Campbell, J. B., Busse, J. W., & Injeyan, H. S. (2000). Chiropractors and vaccination: A historical perspective. Pediatrics, 105(4), e43.

24. Russell, M. L. (2018). The public's perception of chiropractors and immunization. Canadian Medical Association Journal, 190(16), E479.

25. Busse, J. W., Morgan, L., & Campbell, J. B. (2005). Chiropractic antivaccination arguments. Journal of Manipulative and Physiological Therapeutics, 28(5), 367-373.

26. Salsbury, S. A., Goertz, C. M., Twist, E. J., & Lisi, A. J. (2018). Integration of Doctors of Chiropractic Into Private Sector Health Care Facilities in the United States: A Descriptive Survey. Journal of Manipulative and Physiological Therapeutics, 41(2), 149-155.

27. Weeks, W. B., Goertz, C. M., Meeker, W. C., & Marchiori, D. M. (2015). Public Perceptions of Doctors of Chiropractic: Results of a National Survey and Examination of Variation According to Respondents' Likelihood to Use Chiropractic, Experience With Chiropractic, and Chiropractic Supply in Local Health Care Markets. Journal of Manipulative and Physiological Therapeutics, 38(8), 533-544.

28. Foster, N. E., Anema, J. R., Cherkin, D., Chou, R., Cohen, S. P., Gross, D. P., ... & Lancet Low Back Pain Series Working Group. (2018). Prevention and treatment of low back pain: evidence, challenges, and promising directions. The Lancet, 391(10137), 2368-2383.

29. Mior, S., Gamble, B., Barnsley, J., Côté, P., & Côté, E. (2013). Changes in primary care physician's management of low back pain in a model of interprofessional collaborative care: an uncontrolled before-after study. Chiropractic & Manual Therapies, 21(1), 6.

30. Cambron, J. A., Cramer, G. D., & Winterstein, J. (2007). Patient perceptions of chiropractic treatment for primary care disorders. Journal of Manipulative and Physiological Therapeutics, 30(1), 11-16.

31. Schneider, M., Murphy, D., & Hartvigsen, J. (2016). Spine care as a framework for the chiropractic identity. Journal of Chiropractic Humanities, 23(1), 14-21.

32. Johnson, C. (2010). Reflecting on 115 years: the chiropractic profession's philosophical path. Journal of Chiropractic Humanities, 17(1), 1-5.

A Call for Greater Scientific Scrutiny and Public Awareness in Chiropractic Care

As we have explored the complex landscape of chiropractic care, it has become increasingly clear that there is a pressing need for greater scientific scrutiny and public awareness of this profession. While chiropractic has gained significant popularity as a non-invasive treatment option for musculoskeletal conditions [1], it has also been the subject of ongoing controversy and debate regarding its effectiveness, safety, and underlying theories [2]. To ensure that patients receive the highest quality care and to promote the advancement of the profession, it is essential that we prioritize rigorous scientific research and foster open, transparent communication with the public.

One of the primary reasons for the call for greater scientific scrutiny in chiropractic is the need to establish a stronger evidence base for its theories and practices. Despite its long history and widespread use, many of the core concepts in chiropractic, such as the vertebral subluxation complex, remain poorly defined and inadequately supported by scientific evidence [3]. While some studies have suggested that chiropractic interventions, particularly spinal manipulation, may be effective for certain musculoskeletal conditions, the overall quality and consistency of this evidence is limited [4,5]. To build a more solid foundation for the profession, it is crucial that we invest in high-quality research that can help to elucidate the mechanisms of action, optimal treatment parameters, and long-term outcomes of chiropractic care [6].

This research should not only focus on the efficacy of specific interventions but also on the safety and potential risks associated with chiropractic care. While serious adverse events following chiropractic treatments are relatively rare, there have been documented cases of stroke, spinal cord injury, and other complications, particularly in relation to cervical spine manipulation [7,8]. To minimize these risks and ensure patient safety, it is essential that we conduct rigorous studies to identify risk factors, develop evidence-based screening protocols, and establish clear guidelines for informed consent and patient education [9].

In addition to advancing scientific research, there is a critical need for greater public awareness and understanding of chiropractic care. Many patients seek out chiropractic treatment based on anecdotal evidence, personal beliefs, or media portrayals, without a clear understanding of the potential benefits, limitations, and risks [10]. This lack of informed decision-making can lead to unrealistic expectations, delays in seeking necessary medical care, or exposure to unnecessary or inappropriate treatments [11]. To empower patients to make well-informed choices about their health, it is essential that we prioritize public education and outreach efforts that provide accurate, balanced, and evidence-based information about chiropractic care [12].

One key aspect of this public awareness campaign should be to clarify the scope and limitations of chiropractic practice. While some chiropractors may claim to treat a wide range of non-musculoskeletal conditions, such as asthma, allergies, or gastrointestinal disorders, there is little scientific evidence to support these claims [13]. By promoting a more focused and evidence-based scope of practice, centered on the management of musculoskeletal conditions, we can help to reduce confusion and misinformation among the public and foster greater trust and credibility for the profession [14].

Another important component of public awareness is promoting transparency and accountability within the chiropractic profession. Patients have a right to know about the education, training, and licensure requirements for chiropractors, as well as any disciplinary actions or malpractice claims against individual providers [15]. By creating easily accessible and user-friendly resources for patients to research and compare chiropractors, we can help to ensure that they are receiving care from qualified and reputable providers [16].

Greater public awareness can also help to foster more open and collaborative relationships between chiropractors and other healthcare providers. Historically, there has been a degree of tension and mistrust between the chiropractic and medical communities, fueled in part by competing philosophies, professional territoriality, and a lack of interprofessional communication [17]. By promoting a more integrated and patient-centered approach to care, in which chiropractors work collaboratively with primary care physicians, physical therapists, and other providers, we can improve the continuity and quality of care for patients with musculoskeletal conditions [18].

Ultimately, the call for greater scientific scrutiny and public awareness in chiropractic is about prioritizing patient safety, empowerment, and well-being. By investing in rigorous research, promoting evidence-based practice, and fostering open and transparent communication with the public, we can help to ensure that patients receive the highest quality care and achieve the best possible outcomes. This will require a sustained commitment from all stakeholders, including researchers, educators, practitioners, policymakers, and patient advocates, to work together towards a shared vision of a more evidence-based, patient-centered, and integrated approach to chiropractic care.

As we move forward, it is essential that we remain vigilant in our pursuit of scientific truth and public trust. We must be willing to challenge long-held assumptions, to embrace new evidence and insights, and to adapt our practices and policies accordingly. By doing so, we can help to build a stronger, more credible, and more impactful chiropractic profession that truly serves the best interests of patients and society as a whole.

The path ahead may be challenging, but it is also filled with opportunity and promise. By working together, with a shared commitment to scientific excellence, patient-centered care, and public service, we can help to transform the chiropractic profession and improve the lives of countless individuals suffering from musculoskeletal conditions. It is a calling that requires courage, compassion, and a steadfast dedication to the highest principles of healthcare, but it is one that we must embrace if we are to truly realize the potential of chiropractic care in the 21st century.

References

1. Beliveau, P. J., Wong, J. J., Sutton, D. A., Simon, N. B., Bussières, A. E., Mior, S. A., & French, S. D. (2017). The chiropractic profession: a scoping review of utilization rates, reasons for seeking care, patient profiles, and care provided. Chiropractic & Manual Therapies, 25(1), 35.

2. Ernst, E. (2008). Chiropractic: a critical evaluation. Journal of Pain and Symptom Management, 35(5), 544-562.

3. Keating, J. C., Charlton, K. H., Grod, J. P., Perle, S. M., Sikorski, D., & Winterstein, J. F. (2005). Subluxation: dogma or science?. Chiropractic & Osteopathy, 13(1), 17.

4. Bronfort, G., Haas, M., Evans, R., Leininger, B., & Triano, J. (2010). Effectiveness of manual therapies: the UK evidence report. Chiropractic & Osteopathy, 18(1), 3.

5. Goertz, C. M., Long, C. R., Vining, R. D., Pohlman, K. A., Walter, J., & Coulter, I. (2018). Effect of usual medical care plus chiropractic care vs usual medical care alone on pain and disability among US service members with low back pain: a comparative effectiveness clinical trial. JAMA Network Open, 1(1), e180105.

6. Sharma, S., Traeger, A. C., Reed, B., Hamilton, M., O'Connor, D. A., Hoffmann, T. C., ... & Maher, C. G. (2020). Clinician and patient beliefs about diagnostic imaging for low back pain: a systematic qualitative evidence synthesis. BMJ Open, 10(8), e037820.

7. Cassidy, J. D., Boyle, E., Côté, P., He, Y., Hogg-Johnson, S., Silver, F. L., & Bondy, S. J. (2008). Risk of vertebrobasilar stroke and chiropractic care: results of a population-based case-control and case-crossover study. Spine, 33(4S), S176-S183.

8. Gouveia, L. O., Castanho, P., & Ferreira, J. J. (2009). Safety of chiropractic interventions: a systematic review. Spine, 34(11), E405-E413.

9. Stuber, K. J., Wynd, S., & Weis, C. A. (2012). Adverse events from spinal manipulation in the pregnant and postpartum periods: a critical review of the literature. Chiropractic & Manual Therapies, 20(1), 8.

10. Nyiendo, J., Haas, M., & Goodwin, P. (2000). Patient characteristics, practice activities, and one-month outcomes for chronic, recurrent low-back pain treated by chiropractors and family medicine physicians: a practice-based feasibility study. Journal of Manipulative and Physiological Therapeutics, 23(4), 239-245.

11. Walker, B. F., French, S. D., Grant, W., & Green, S. (2010). Combined chiropractic interventions for low-back pain. Cochrane Database of Systematic Reviews, (4).

12. Cambron, J. A., Cramer, G. D., & Winterstein, J. (2007). Patient perceptions of chiropractic treatment for primary care disorders. Journal of Manipulative and Physiological Therapeutics, 30(1), 11-16.

13. Ernst, E. (2009). Chiropractic treatment for gastrointestinal problems: a systematic review of clinical trials. Canadian Journal of Gastroenterology, 23(6), 475-478.

14. Schneider, M., Murphy, D., & Hartvigsen, J. (2016). Spine care as a framework for the chiropractic identity. Journal of Chiropractic Humanities, 23(1), 14-21.

15. Shaw, L., Descarreaux, M., Bryans, R., Duranleau, M., Marcoux, H., Potter, B., ... & White, E. (2010). A systematic review of chiropractic management of adults with Whiplash-Associated Disorders: recommendations for advancing evidence-based practice and research. Work, 35(3), 369-394.

16. Puhl, A. A., Reinhart, C. J., Doan, J. B., & Vernon, H. (2017). The quality of placebos used in randomized, controlled trials of lumbar and pelvic joint thrust manipulation—a systematic review. The Spine Journal, 17(3), 445-456.

17. McGregor, M., Puhl, A. A., Reinhart, C., Injeyan, H. S., & Soave, D. (2014). Differentiating intraprofessional attitudes toward paradigms in health care delivery among chiropractic factions: results from a randomly sampled survey. BMC Complementary and Alternative Medicine, 14(1), 51.

18. Salsbury, S. A., Goertz, C. M., Twist, E. J., & Lisi, A. J. (2018). Integration of doctors of chiropractic into private sector health care facilities in the United States: a descriptive survey. Journal of Manipulative and Physiological Therapeutics, 41(2), 149-155.

Prioritizing Evidence-Based Care: A Call to Action for Chiropractic Patients and Providers

As we conclude our exploration of the chiropractic landscape, it is crucial to emphasize the importance of evidence-based care in ensuring the best possible outcomes for patients. Throughout this journey, we have encountered a complex tapestry of historical controversies, theoretical debates, and varying practice approaches within the chiropractic profession [1]. However, amidst this diversity, one fundamental principle should guide both patients and providers in their pursuit of optimal musculoskeletal health: a steadfast commitment to evidence-based care.

Evidence-based care refers to the conscientious, explicit, and judicious use of the best available scientific evidence in making decisions about the care of individual patients [2]. This approach integrates clinical expertise, patient values and preferences, and the most up-to-date research findings to inform healthcare decision-making [3]. By prioritizing evidence-based care, patients and providers can work together to ensure that chiropractic interventions are safe, effective, and aligned with the latest scientific understanding of musculoskeletal conditions.

For patients seeking chiropractic care, embracing an evidence-based approach means becoming active, informed participants in their own healthcare decisions. This involves asking questions, expressing preferences and concerns, and critically evaluating the information provided by chiropractors and other sources [4]. Patients should feel empowered to inquire about the evidence supporting proposed treatments, the potential risks and benefits, and the availability of alternative options [5]. By engaging in open, collaborative dialogue with their chiropractors, patients can make well-informed decisions that align with their values, goals, and unique clinical circumstances.

To support evidence-based decision-making, patients are encouraged to seek out reliable, trustworthy sources of information about chiropractic care. These may include reputable healthcare

organizations, government health agencies, and peer-reviewed scientific journals [6]. Patients should be cautious of anecdotal evidence, testimonials, or unsubstantiated claims, as these may not accurately reflect the true benefits and risks of chiropractic interventions [7]. By accessing high-quality, evidence-based information, patients can better understand their condition, evaluate treatment options, and engage in meaningful discussions with their healthcare providers.

For chiropractors, prioritizing evidence-based care requires a commitment to lifelong learning, critical thinking, and a willingness to adapt practice patterns in light of new research findings [8]. This means staying up-to-date with the latest scientific literature, attending continuing education courses, and participating in professional networks that promote evidence-based practice [9]. Chiropractors should be well-versed in the principles of clinical research, able to critically appraise the quality and relevance of scientific studies, and skilled in applying this knowledge to individual patient care [10].

Evidence-based chiropractic care also demands a patient-centered approach that respects individual preferences, needs, and values [11]. Chiropractors should engage in shared decision-making with their patients, openly discussing the strengths and limitations of different treatment options and collaboratively developing care plans that align with patients' goals and expectations [12]. This approach fosters trust, transparency, and a therapeutic alliance that can enhance patient satisfaction, adherence, and clinical outcomes [13].

Furthermore, evidence-based chiropractic care necessitates a commitment to interprofessional collaboration and communication [14]. Chiropractors should work closely with primary care physicians, physical therapists, and other healthcare providers to ensure coordinated, comprehensive care for patients with musculoskeletal conditions [15]. By fostering open dialogue, mutual respect, and a shared focus on patient well-being, chiropractors can contribute to a more integrated, patient-centered healthcare system that delivers high-quality, evidence-based care [16].

Prioritizing evidence-based care also requires a willingness to confront and address practices or beliefs within the chiropractic profession that may not align with current scientific evidence. This includes re-evaluating the role of traditional chiropractic theories, such as vertebral subluxation, in light of modern research findings [17]. It also means being transparent about the limitations and uncertainties of certain chiropractic interventions and avoiding overstating their benefits or indications [18]. By embracing a culture of scientific rigor, self-reflection, and continuous quality improvement, the chiropractic profession can strengthen its credibility, trust, and impact within the broader healthcare landscape [19].

Ultimately, the call to prioritize evidence-based care in chiropractic is a call to action for patients, providers, and the profession as a whole. It is a recognition that the pursuit of optimal musculoskeletal health requires a shared commitment to scientific truth, patient empowerment, and collaborative, patient-centered care. By aligning chiropractic practice with the best available evidence, we can unlock the full potential of this unique and valuable healthcare discipline, improving the lives of countless individuals suffering from musculoskeletal conditions.

As readers of this book, you have a powerful opportunity to shape the future of chiropractic care by prioritizing evidence-based approaches in your own healthcare decisions and interactions. Whether you are a patient seeking care for a musculoskeletal condition, a chiropractor striving to deliver the highest quality care, or a healthcare provider collaborating with chiropractors in patient management, your commitment to evidence-based practice can make a meaningful difference. By asking questions, staying informed, and advocating for science-based care, you can contribute to a healthcare system that truly puts patients first and optimizes health outcomes for all.

So let us move forward together, armed with knowledge, compassion, and a steadfast dedication to evidence-based chiropractic care. By prioritizing science, empowering patients, and fostering collaboration, we can transform the chiropractic profession and the lives of those it serves, one patient at a time. The journey may be challenging, but the rewards – improved health, reduced suf-

fering, and a more patient-centered, integrated healthcare system – are well worth the effort. Let us embrace this call to action and work together to build a brighter, more evidence-based future for chiropractic care.

References

1. Johnson, C. (2010). Reflecting on 115 years: the chiropractic profession's philosophical path. Journal of Chiropractic Humanities, 17(1), 1-5.
2. Sackett, D. L., Rosenberg, W. M., Gray, J. M., Haynes, R. B., & Richardson, W. S. (1996). Evidence based medicine: what it is and what it isn't. BMJ, 312(7023), 71-72.
3. Straus, S. E., Glasziou, P., Richardson, W. S., & Haynes, R. B. (2018). Evidence-based medicine e-book: How to practice and teach EBM. Elsevier Health Sciences.
4. Stacey, D., Légaré, F., Lewis, K., Barry, M. J., Bennett, C. L., Eden, K. B., ... & Trevena, L. (2017). Decision aids for people facing health treatment or screening decisions. Cochrane Database of Systematic Reviews, (4).
5. Hoffmann, T. C., Montori, V. M., & Del Mar, C. (2014). The connection between evidence-based medicine and shared decision making. JAMA, 312(13), 1295-1296.
6. Dagenais, S., & Haldeman, S. (2012). Evidence-based management of low back pain. Elsevier Health Sciences.
7. Chou, R., Deyo, R., Friedly, J., Skelly, A., Hashimoto, R., Weimer, M., ... & Brodt, E. D. (2017). Nonpharmacologic therapies for low back pain: a systematic review for an American College of Physicians clinical practice guideline. Annals of Internal Medicine, 166(7), 493-505.
8. Bussieres, A. E., Al Zoubi, F., Stuber, K., French, S. D., Boruff, J., Corrigan, J., & Thomas, A. (2016). Evidence-based practice, research utilization, and knowledge translation in chiropractic: a scoping review. BMC Complementary and Alternative Medicine, 16(1), 216.
9. Schneider, M. J., Evans, R., Haas, M., Leach, M., Hawk, C., Long, C., ... & Terhorst, L. (2015). US chiropractors' attitudes, skills and use of evidence-based practice: A cross-sectional national survey. Chiropractic & Manual Therapies, 23(1), 16.
10. Halloun, H., & Cawston, H. (2021). A practical approach to evidence-based chiropractic: Acquiring the skill of efficiently locating, appraising, and applying scientific evidence in clinical practice. Journal of Chiropractic Education.
11. Salsbury, S. A., Goertz, C. M., Twist, E. J., & Lisi, A. J. (2018). Integration of doctors of chiropractic into private sector health care facilities in the United States: a descriptive survey. Journal of Manipulative and Physiological Therapeutics, 41(2), 149-155.
12. Goertz, C. M., Salsbury, S. A., Long, C. R., Vining, R. D., Andresen, A. A., Hondras, M. A., ... & Wallace, R. B. (2017). Patient-centered professional practice models for managing low back pain in older adults: a pilot randomized controlled trial. BMC Geriatrics, 17(1), 235.
13. Haas, M., Vavrek, D., Peterson, D., Polissar, N., & Neradilek, M. B. (2014). Dose-response and efficacy of spinal manipulation for care of chronic low back pain: a randomized controlled trial. The Spine Journal, 14(7), 1106-1116.
14. Weeks, W. B., Goertz, C. M., Meeker, W. C., & Marchiori, D. M. (2015). Public perceptions of doctors of chiropractic: results of a national survey and examination of variation according to respondents' likelihood to use chiropractic, experience with chiropractic, and chiropractic supply in local health care markets. Journal of Manipulative and Physiological Therapeutics, 38(8), 533-544.
15. Lisi, A. J., Salsbury, S. A., Hawk, C., Vining, R. D., Wallace, R. B., Branson, R., ... & Goertz, C. M. (2018). Chiropractic integrated care pathway for low back pain in veterans: results of a Delphi consensus process. Journal of Manipulative and Physiological Therapeutics, 41(2), 137-148.

16. Salsbury, S. A., Vining, R. D., Hartvigsen, J., Dong, W., Lisi, A. J., Deyo, R. A., ... & Goertz, C. M. (2020). Development and pilot testing of an interprofessional collaboration model for chiropractic, medical, and physical therapy students: The Interprofessional Model for Management of Musculoskeletal and other Ambulatory Care Conditions. Journal of Interprofessional Care, 1-9.
17. Keating, J. C., Charlton, K. H., Grod, J. P., Perle, S. M., Sikorski, D., & Winterstein, J. F. (2005). Subluxation: dogma or science?. Chiropractic & Osteopathy, 13(1), 17.
18. Walker, B. F., Armson, A., Hodgetts, C., Jacques, A., Chin, F. E., Kow, G., ... & Wright, A. (2017). Knowledge, attitude, influences and use of complementary and alternative medicine (CAM) among chiropractic and nursing students. Chiropractic & Manual Therapies, 25(1), 29.
19. Murphy, D. R., Schneider, M. J., Seaman, D. R., Perle, S. M., & Nelson, C. F. (2008). How can chiropractic become a respected mainstream profession? The example of podiatry. Chiropractic & Osteopathy, 16(1), 10.